Mariem Nouira
Nesrine Souayeh
Mohamed Maatouk

Healthcare-associated infections:

Mariem Nouira
Nesrine Souayeh
Mohamed Maatouk

Healthcare-associated infections:

Background and protocol for a study estimating the incidence and additional medical costs in hospitals

ScienciaScripts

Cover image: www.ingimage.com

This book is a translation from the original published under ISBN 978-620-6-72124-6.

Publisher:
Sciencia Scripts
is a trademark of
Dodo Books Indian Ocean Ltd. and OmniScriptum S.R.L publishing group

120 High Road, East Finchley, London, N2 9ED, United Kingdom
Str. Armeneasca 28/1, office 1, Chisinau MD-2012, Republic of Moldova, Europe
Printed at: see last page
ISBN: 978-620-8-32972-3

Contents

Resume

Introduction:

Healthcare-associated infections (HAIs) are a major global public health concern, and our aim was to provide an update on HAIs and to develop an example of a protocol for an incidence survey and an approach to extra costs in hospitals.

Methods:

A bibliographical review of the literature was carried out in order to provide a theoretical background and develop a protocol.

Results:

This is a cohort study protocol with prospective data collection. To estimate incidence, we used 3 epidemiological indicators: cumulative incidence, incidence density and medical device exposure ratio.

To assess the cost of HCAI, we looked at the direct medical costs associated with longer hospital stays (comparing infected cases with uninfected controls), as well as the costs associated with the use of antibiotics to treat these infections.

Conclusion:A method for regular monitoring of the incidence and cost of these infections must be introduced in each hospital establishment for effective control.

I. Introduction

Healthcare-associated infections (HAIs) contracted in hospitals are also known as nosocomial infections (NIs). They represent a major public health concern worldwide, with a heavy burden of attributable morbidity and mortality [1,2,3].

This prolongs the length of time patients spend in care, thereby increasing the cost of treatment and care [4].

According to the Center for Disease Prevention and Control (CDC), they are the leading cause of avoidable death and disability in hospital patients [5].

According to a recent literature review by the European Centre for Disease Prevention and Control (ECDC), more than 3.2 million patients contract at least one HCAI each year in European countries, resulting in 16 million additional hospital days and 37,000 attributable deaths [6].

According to the World Health Organisation (WHO), the additional annual financial losses due to HAIs were estimated at between 13 and 24 billion euros [7].

In developing countries, the burden of NI is considerably higher than in developed countries, with an estimated overall prevalence of 15.5 per 100 patients [8].

According to the WHO, the risk of contracting an IN is multiplied by 2 to 20 times in developing countries, with a prevalence that can exceed 25% in some countries [9].

This problem is still largely underestimated, given the paucity of data and epidemiological studies [10].

Tunisia has not been spared by this scourge, which is constantly increasing and placing a heavy burden on the health system. So far, two national surveys of the prevalence of nosocomial infections have been carried out. The first was carried out in 2005 ("NosoTun-2005") and showed a prevalence of 6.6% [11]. The second and most recent survey ("NosoTun-2012") showed a national prevalence of infected patients of 6.7% (IC95%: 6.2%-7.3%) and a prevalence of nosocomial infections of 7.7% (IC95%: 7.2%-8.3%) [12].

According to a multicentre survey that was conducted in 2017 in all medical resuscitation departments in Tunisia, more than one in four patients had an IN on the day of the survey [13].

Another survey was recently carried out at the Charles Nicolle Hospital in Tunis (HCN) and found a fairly high overall prevalence of IN, estimated at 13.8% (95% CI: 10.0% -17.6%).

II. Issues

Surveillance of nosocomial infections is recognised as an essential and fundamental step in the fight against these infections [14].

It must be an integral part of any infection prevention and control policy in order to improve the quality and safety of care in healthcare establishments [15,16.17].

Setting up a system to monitor hospital-acquired infections is a vital and essential activity. It makes it possible to take stock of the problem being monitored (quantify the extent of the problem and study its trend) in order to identify and determine priorities, target actions to be taken, guide prevention activities and generate a health policy commitment [15].

Surveillance data therefore represent the key indicators and benchmarks needed to manage the risk of nosocomial infections effectively, and which can be used to monitor and evaluate the extent to which a prevention programme is being implemented [14,18,17].

Different monitoring methodologies can be adopted. Each approach differs according to the time required to carry it out, the human and material resources available and the expected objective [19].

Two main methods can be recommended for carrying out surveillance surveys for nosocomial infections:

- Prevalence studies (one-off or cross-cutting) :

They are based on a one-off collection of data, at a given time (on a given day), on the infectious situation of each patient. They can be carried out at regular intervals, such as the annual prevalence surveys for nosocomial infections [14]. This surveillance method has the advantage of being quick to carry out, easy to implement and supervise, and less costly, with a less cumbersome methodological approach than other incidence surveys.

In fact, prevalence surveys have been found to be useful and cost-effective in terms of saving time and estimating the extent of NI, particularly in hospitals with limited resources [20,21,22,23].

On the other hand, they have the disadvantage of not being able to identify new infections occurring outside the survey period, and of not being able to estimate the real risk of these infections given that there is no patient follow-up [19].

- Incidence studies (longitudinal) :

Although they are costly and demanding in terms of the time and resources required [24], they are considered to be the most scientifically valid reference method (the gold standard) for infection control. They are based on a rigorous methodology with continuous monitoring of hospitalised patients over time. They consist of prospectively recording and detecting, as and when they occur, all new cases of infection occurring during hospitalisation [14]. They provide a precise measure of the risk of contracting an infection and identify the main risk factors involved. They are particularly recommended in high-risk infection specialties such as intensive care and neonatology [19,24,25].

In addition, the problem of the extra cost and economic impact of these infections is making the situation worse and worse [26]. Given the extent of this burden in

Tunisia, with a non-negligible prevalence of nosocomial infections in healthcare establishments [12], as well as the serious subsequent complications, a study of the economic impact of nosocomial infections is necessary and of considerable importance. This will enable us to draw up an up-to-date inventory of the situation in terms of cost, and to highlight the major economic impact of these infections in our country. These data will enable us to orientate preventive actions and guide health policies and decision-making concerning investment in the fight against these infections [27].

In view of the foregoing, conducting a survey of the incidence and estimation of the extra cost of HAIs in Tunisian healthcare establishments is essential and of capital importance. However, before carrying out this type of survey, a review of the literature and a bibliographic synthesis on this subject based on a selection of relevant scientific articles is an essential and indispensable step. This will enable us to build up a state of the art with a targeted, in-depth and critical study of existing work carried out in the field of our research, both in Tunisia and internationally.

With this in mind, we propose in this work:

- firstly, to provide an update on the various surveys of the incidence and cost of NI at national and international level
- secondly, to draw up an example protocol for a survey of the incidence and evaluation of additional costs in the surgical and intensive care environment at the Charles Nicolle Hospital in Tunis (HCN).

III. Theoretical background on IAS

1. History

The term "nosocomial" has been in use since the 18th century, and has its origins in ancient Greece:

Etymologically, *"Nosos"* means disease and "*Komein*" means to care for, which forms the word "*nosocomiale*", care given to the sick [28].

The history of hospital-acquired infections and hygiene in general has been marked by a number of key players. They are shown in Figure 1.

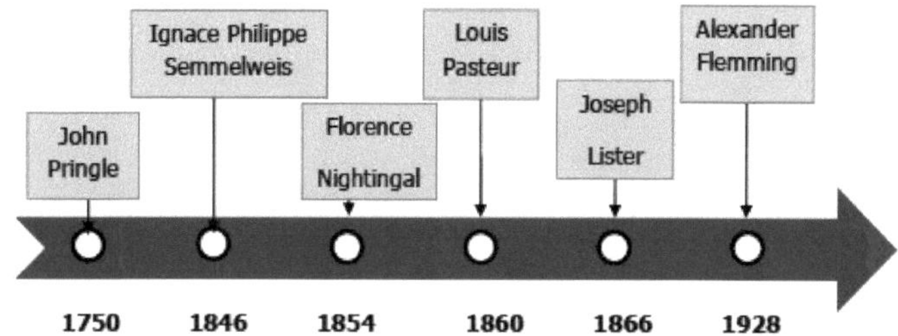

Ranking of substances antiseptics	Evidence of the importance hand washing for staff	Nursing care from soldiers in the Crimean War	Discover microbes and introduction to wound asepsis	Use of acid phenique as a basis for surgical asepsis	Discover the penicillin

Figure 1: Historical chronological review of the main key players who contributed to the development of the principle of hygiene and the fight against IN. In 1750, the Scottish surgeon John Pringle (1707-1782) made his first observations on "hospital-acquired infections" and identified and classified antiseptic substances[29].

From the 19th century onwards, increasing urbanisation and scientific progress led to the development of hospital hygiene:

Ignace Philippe Semmelweis (1818-1865) was a Hungarian obstetrician who was the first to advocate the importance of hand hygiene in preventing hospital infections. In 1846, in a maternity ward at the Vienna Hospital, he observed a high mortality rate from puerperal fever among parturient women who had been delivered by medical students who had gone from the autopsy room to the maternity ward without washing their hands. He then made hand washing compulsory for nursing staff by using a dilute chloride of lime-based antiseptic solution between two acts of care. He thus demonstrated the importance and usefulness of hand washing after observing a considerable drop in the mortality rate from puerperal fever, from 18% to less than 3% [30,31] (Figures 2 and 3).

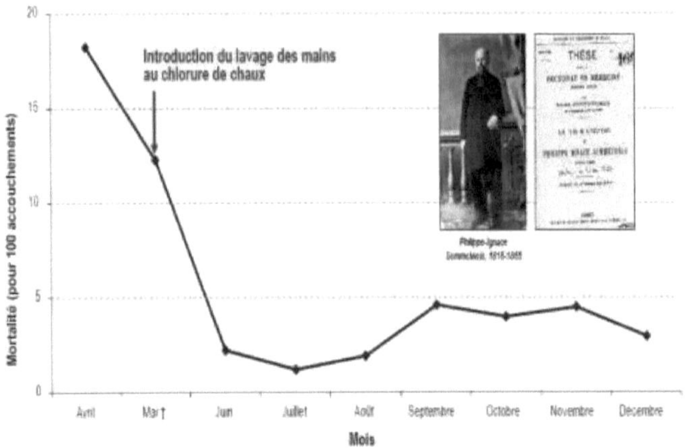

Figure 2: Trends in maternal mortality due to puerperal fever, Vienna Hospital Maternity Ward, Pavilion I, April to December 1847.

Ignace Philippe
Semmelweis

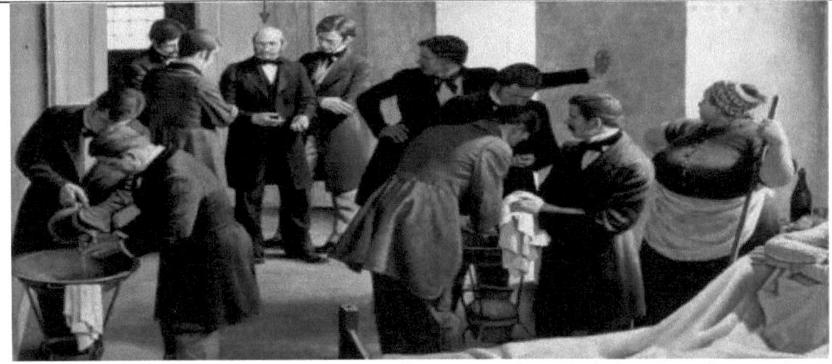

Figure 3. View of a delivery room at the Vienna hospital showing Semmelweis teaching hand hygiene to students.

- Florence Nightingale (1820 - 1910), an English nurse, was considered a pioneer of modern nursing and hospital hygiene. She introduced the use of statistics applied to the medical field and invented pie charts to explain the causes of soldiers' deaths in the Crimean War (1854).
- In 1860, Louis Pasteur (1822-1895), the protagonist of microbiology, discovered the existence of microbes and advocated the development of asepsis rules in healthcare, especially for wounds [32].
- In 1866, Joseph Lister, an English surgeon, proposed the use of phenic acid as a basis for asepsis in wounds and surgical procedures.

In the 20th century, Alexander Flemming (1881-1955), a Scottish microbiologist renowned for his interest in combating infectious diseases, discovered penicillin in

1928.

2. Update and new definitions

Initially, the scope of the definition of NI was limited to the hospital environment.

A nosocomial infection is therefore any infection contracted during a stay in a healthcare establishment (hospital, clinic, etc.) or from any other procedure carried out in hospital, and must be clinically and microbiologically identifiable [28]. According to the Committee of Ministers of the Council of Europe, a nosocomial infection is "any clinically/microbiologically recognisable disease due to micro-organisms contracted in hospital, which affects either the patient as a result of his activity or not, while the patient is in hospital" [33].

This definition has become unsuited to current healthcare practices. Whether an infection is nosocomial or community-acquired used to be judged solely on the basis of where the infection was acquired. In recent years, the multiplication of care pathways, such as the diversification of care structures, the multiplication of care providers, and even the sometimes late onset of infection after surgery, have led to changes in certain definitions being taken into account and have resulted in the definitions being updated [28].

The concept of nosocomial infections was updated in November 2007 by the Comité Technique des Infections Nosocomiales et des Infections Liees aux Soins (CTINILS) [28], and they have now been included more generally within HCAIs. The broadened concept of HCAIs now covers infectious episodes resulting from healthcare acts, regardless of where the care is provided or delivered (healthcare establishment, outpatient care, home, private practice, etc.) and encompassing, in the broadest sense, all types of healthcare services, whether for diagnostic, therapeutic, screening or primary prevention purposes [34].

The term "associated" with care is a neutral term that does not imply causality.

General definition of IAS

"An infection is said to be associated with care if it occurs during or at the end of a patient's care (diagnostic, therapeutic, palliative, preventive or educational), and if it was neither present nor incubating at the start of the care. When the state of infection at the start of care is not known precisely, a period of at least 48 hours or a period longer than the incubation period is commonly accepted to define an HCAI. However, it is recommended that the plausibility of the association between the treatment and the infection be assessed in each case.

For surgical site infections

"Infections occurring within 30 days of the operation or, if an implant, prosthesis or prosthetic device is used, within one year of the operation, are usually considered to be associated with care. However, whatever the delay, it is recommended that the plausibility of the association between the operation and the infection be assessed in each case, taking into account the type of germ involved.

A nosocomial infection is an HCAI contracted in a healthcare establishment

The figure below shows the evolution of IAS appointments over the years:

(figure 4)

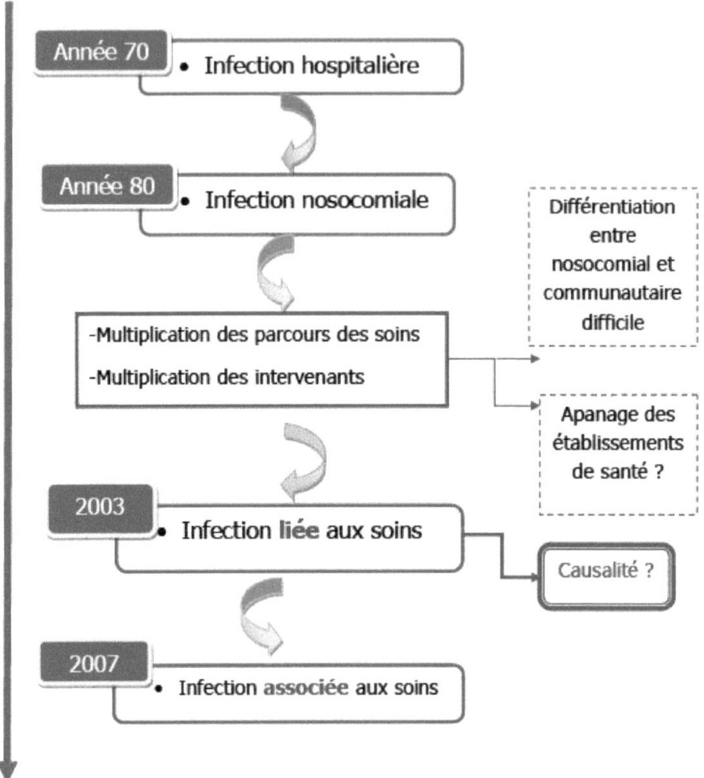

Figure 4: Chronology of IAS appointments

3. Origins and transmission routes of HCAIs

In general, an infection can be caused by :

- Germs hosted by the patient himself: the infection is said to be ENDOGENIC
- Micro-organisms from the contaminated environment (contaminated inanimate elements or human beings): the infection is said to be EXOGENOUS.

More precisely, we can distinguish four categories of origin (reservoirs) responsible for HCAIs:

3.1 The patient's own commensal flora

There are 3 main types of commensal flora: cutaneous, respiratory and digestive. There are 2 types of cutaneous flora:

- Transient flora, which is a sign of transient contamination and is easily eliminated by simply washing the hands with soap.
- A protective resident flora that forms a veritable bacterial barrier, reinforcing the individual's immune defences by protecting against potentially pathogenic germs.

Digestive or faecal flora can be formidable if found in a hospital ward, if basic

hygiene precautions are not followed.
The patient's usual flora undergoes qualitative changes during the first 5 days of hospitalisation. Following certain invasive procedures, these germs may be moved from a place where they are harmless to another where they multiply differently and become pathogenic. Certain germs in the hospital environment (Gram-negative bacilli, anaerobes, etc.) can replace the commensal flora and colonise a number of sites (pulmonary, blood, urinary, operative, catheter), which can cause infections under certain conditions (immunodepression, virulence of germs, etc.).
The entry points may be mucous membrane lesions or skin lesions (wounds, burns, skin diseases, etc.).
o In this case, the route of transmission is called : Auto-infection (figure 5).

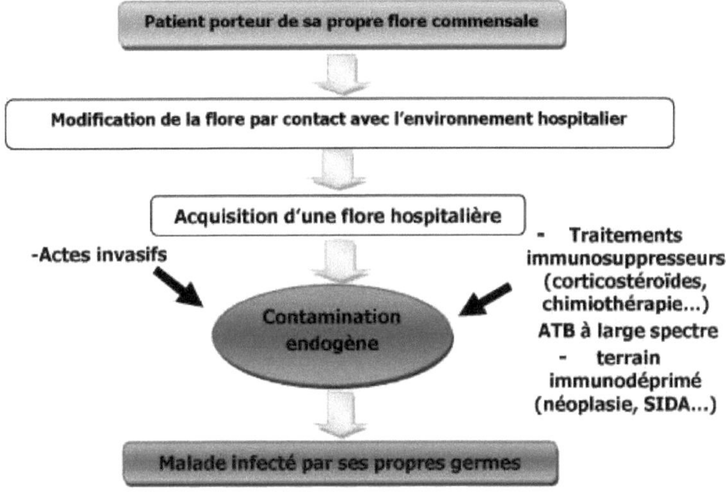

Figure 5. Schématisation du mécanisme de contamination endogène

3.2 Nursing, medical and paramedical staff

It may be colonised or infected either by the environment or contaminated equipment, or by another colonised or infected patient.
Healthcare staff are a key factor in the spread of HCAIs.
o In this case, the transmission route is said to be: Xeno-infection

3.3 The patient infects or simply colonises

In this case, the germ responsible for the HCAI comes from another patient. Transmission is most often carried out by healthcare staff working with several patients, spreading germs from one person to another.
These infections are known as "cross infections".
This factor is just as important as the nursing staff.
o In this case, the transmission route is said to be : Hetero-infection

3.4 The environment

It is represented by inanimate objects such as :

- floors, objects, surfaces, washbasins, ambient air, food, etc.
- medical devices: mainly intra-vascular monitoring and respiratory assistance equipment...

It can be contaminated by the patient or by healthcare staff.

In a strategy to prevent and combat HCAIs, the environment plays a less decisive role than other factors.

In this case, the route of transmission is called exo-infection (Figure 6).

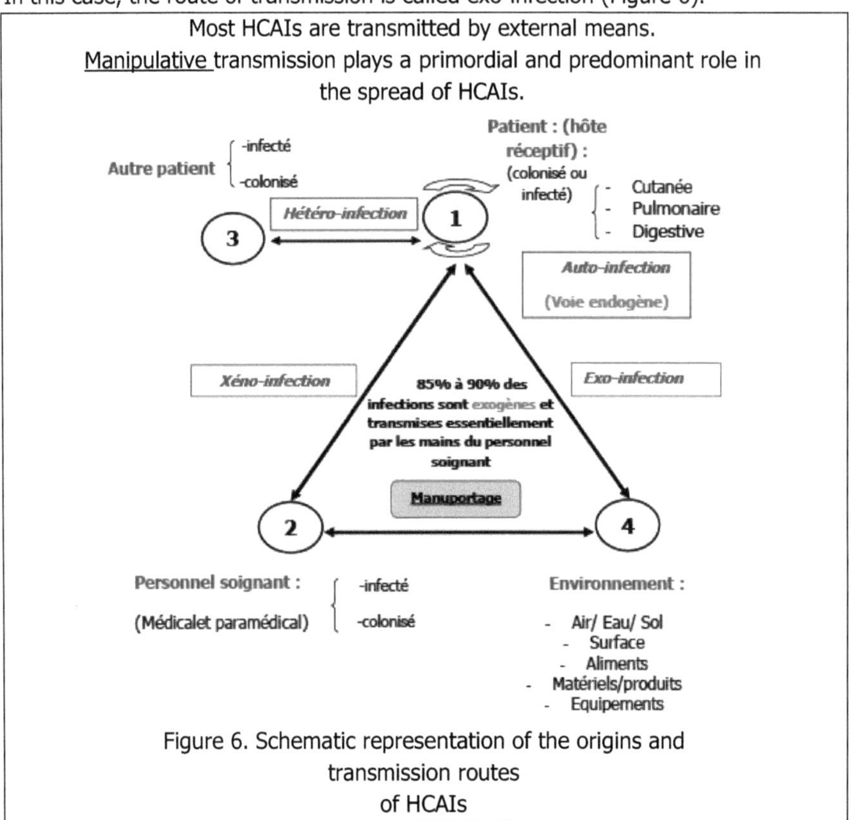

Figure 6. Schematic representation of the origins and transmission routes of HCAIs

4. IAS risk factors

The occurrence of HCAIs is favoured by several risk factors, which may be : - Healthcare-associated: essentially the acquisition of infections directly linked to healthcare procedures through the use of invasive procedures.

- Lies to the patient: immune status, terrain, susceptibility...
- Lies to the excessive and irrational use of antibiotics
- The organisation of care (resources available, staff training, etc.)
- Lies to the care environment: design, quality, maintenance.

4.1 Invasive techniques

They represent the main risk factor for HAIs.

They mainly concern venous and arterial catheterisation, intubation and mechanical ventilation, urinary catheterisation and many others (endoscopy, dialysis, punctures, infusions, drainage, parental feeding, etc.).

The risk of infection is linked to :

- Insertion site: risk of perineal contamination for the inferior vena cava. Preference should be given to catheterisation of the superior vena cava.
- The implementation period
- The frequency and multiplication of manipulations.

According to the latest French national survey on the prevalence of nosocomial infections in healthcare establishments, which was carried out in 2017 [35], the prevalence of infected patients and nosocomial infections was significantly higher in patients exposed to medical devices (MDs), mainly vascular catheters, urinary catheters and respiratory assistance. The risk was 4.5 times higher for patients with an indwelling medical device on the day of the survey than for those without (Figure 7).

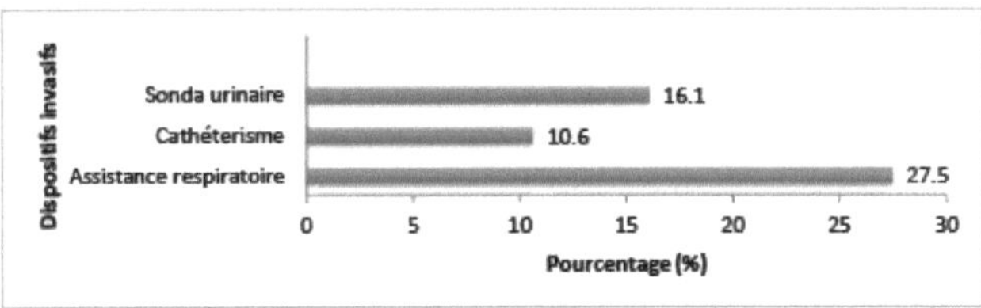

Figure 7. Bar chart representing the frequency of exposure of infected patients to invasive devices. National prevalence survey, France, 2017.

According to the latest Tunisian national survey of the prevalence of nosocomial infections, "NosoTun 2012" [12]: the multivariate analysis showed that the nosocomial risk was multiplied by 5.3 in the case of suprapubic puncture, by 3.8 in the presence of a central vascular catheterism (CVC), by 2.3 in the presence of a urinary catheter, by 1.9 in the case of intubation/ventilation and by 1.8 in the presence of a peripheral vascular catheterism (CVP).

A recent prevalence survey conducted in 2018 at the HCN in Tunis showed that the prevalence of infected patients was significantly higher among those with at least one DM during the 7 days prior to the survey compared with patients without an invasive device (26.7% versus 5.9%; $p < 10^{-3}$). The prevalence of infected patients increased with the number of DMs (Figure 8).

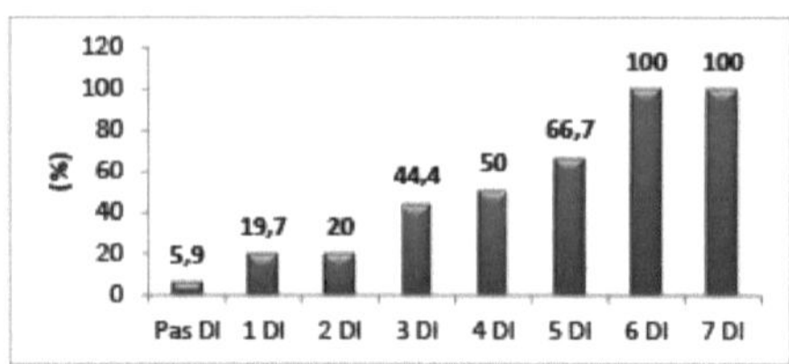

Figure 8. Prevalence of infected patients according to the number of IDs, prevalence survey at HCN Tunis, 2018

4.2 The irrational use of ATBs

The notion of irrational use of ATBs encompasses several situations: excessive treatment of benign diseases, misuse of ATBs, excessive use of injections, self-medication, and premature discontinuation of treatment [36]. This factor is considered to be one of the main causes of HCAI.

Unnecessary overuse of ATBs accelerates the phenomenon of resistance. It leads to the selection of resistant bacteria in the hospital environment, which may even become multi-resistant [37].

According to the WHO, almost half of all drug prescriptions are unjustified and misused, posing a major threat to both health and the economy. In fact, inappropriate prescribing of ATBs can cause undesirable events that can lead to prolonged illness or even death [36].

4.3 Patient's condition

The risk of contracting an HCAI is increased by :

- Age (>45 years) [38].
- The severity of the condition requiring hospitalisation (polytrauma, burns, acute visceral failure, etc.)
- Chronic diseases (diabetes, renal failure, liver failure, heart failure, etc.) [39]
- Immunosuppressive therapy

4.4 Others

There are other factors that increase the risk of developing HAIs. These include

-The architecture of the premises does not allow infected patients to be isolated

- Insufficient training in hospital hygiene for nursing staff
- The nature of the department's activity. Certain departments are considered to be high-risk, such as intensive care and infectious diseases departments.
- Poorly organised care
- Overcrowding in hospital departments

5. Microorganisms responsible for HAIs

HCAIs are often caused by undesirable germs (viruses, bacteria, fungi, parasites) that belong to the hospital flora (Figure 9).

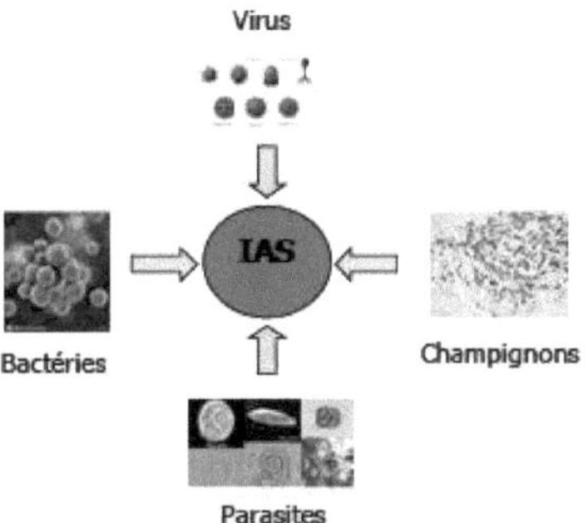

Figure 9. The different types of germs responsible for HCAIs

Bacteria are responsible for around 90% of HCAIs [40] .

Overall, gram-negative bacilli account for 60% of germs reported in European series [41].

According to the Institut national de la sante et de la recherche medicale (Inserm) in France, three main bacteria are responsible for more than half of all cases of nosocomial infections: Escherichia coli, *Staphylococcus aureus* and *Pseudomonas Aeruginosa* [42].

According to the results of the latest national survey on the prevalence of nosocomial infections carried out in France in 2017, the most frequently isolated bacterial families were, in descending order: enterobacteria, with a relative share of 43.8%, followed by gram-positive cocci in 34.2% of cases and gram-negative bacilli other than enterobacteria in 9.8% of cases [35].

Escherichia coli was the most commonly identified germ in almost a quarter of cases (Figure 10).

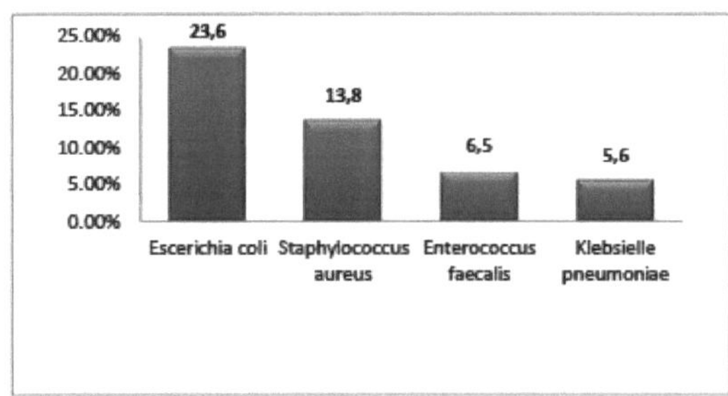

Figure 10. Proportional distribution of the most frequently frequently identified. National survey on the prevalence of nosocomial infections, France, 2017

In Tunisia, according to the latest national prevalence survey carried out in 2012 ("NosoTun2012"), the most common germs responsible for nosocomial infections *were Klebsiela pneumoniae, Pseudomonas Aeruginosa* and *Escherichia coli* [12] (Figure 11).

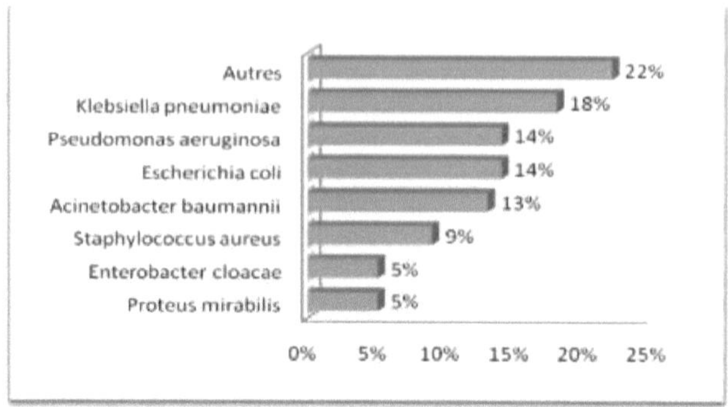

Figure 11. Proportional distribution of germs identified. National prevalence survey, NosoTun 2012

Another NI prevalence survey was conducted in 2018 at HCN. *LE.* Coliet le *Pseudomonas Aeroginosa* were the most common germs (Figure 12).

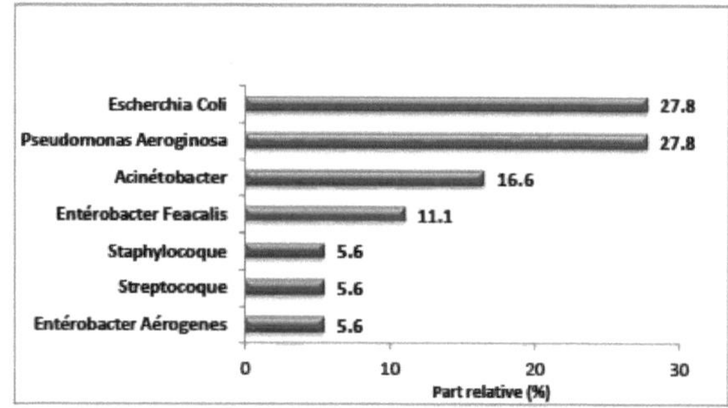

Figure 12. Proportional distribution of germs identified. IN prevalence survey, HCN Tunis, 2018.

In medical intensive care settings, according to a recent multicentre Tunisian survey of the prevalence of nosocomial infections carried out in 2017, the most commonly identified germs were *Pseudomonas aeroginosa* and *Klebsiela pneumoniae* [13].

6. Antibiotic resistance

Germ resistance to ATBs is a major health issue, leading to an increase in mortality and longer hospital stays, with additional financial costs for healthcare establishments [43]. Multi-resistant organisms account for 25% of HAIs worldwide [44]. According to the WHO, the number of deaths attributable to bacterial resistance is estimated at 700,000 per year [45].

Each time, bacteria develop new resistance mechanisms following an accumulation of natural resistances (forming an integral part of the genetic capital of a bacterial species) and acquired resistances (secondary to chromosomal mutations or, more frequently, to the acquisition of resistance genes carried by mobile genetic elements that can spread very easily from one bacterium to another) (figure 13) [37,46].

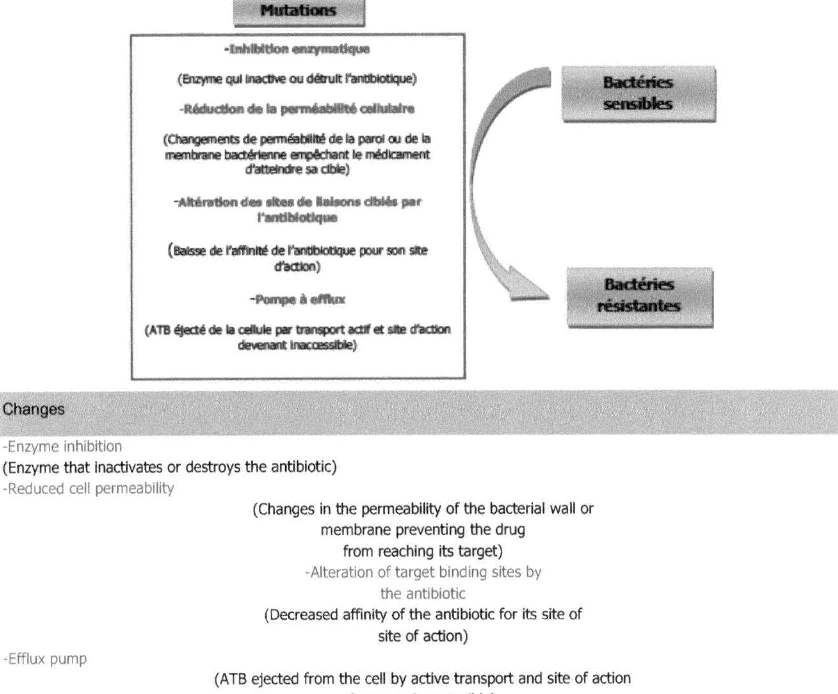

Figure 13. Summary diagram of the phenomenon of resistance and its main main mechanisms

Multi-drug resistant bacteria (MDRB) are defined by a phenotype combining resistance to several drugs that can compromise therapeutic possibilities. The emergence of this phenomenon has become a major global health concern.

It is mainly the result of the massive and often inappropriate use of ATBs.

Many factors and situations can contribute to the emergence and spread of this phenomenon. They are shown in the following diagram (Figure 14) [47] :

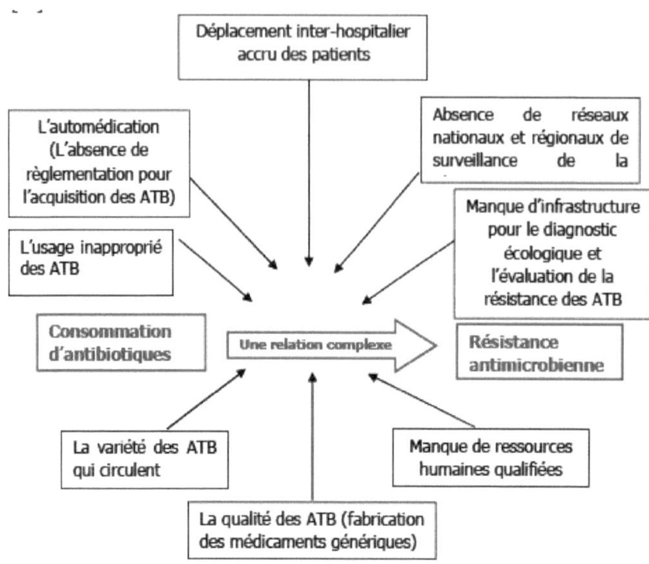

Increased patient movement between hospitals
Lack of national and regional resistance surveillance networks Lack of infrastructure for ecological diagnosis and assessment of ATB resistance
Self-medication (absence of regulations governing the purchase of ATBs)
Inappropriate use of ATBs
Antibiotic consumption
Antimicrobial resistance
A complex relationship
The variety of ATBs in circulation
Lack of qualified human resources
Quality of ATBs (manufacture of generic medicines)

Figure 14. Main factors involved in the emergence of antibiotic resistance

In France, *meticilino-resistant* strains *of Staphylococcus aureus* (MRSA) are the most common type of MRB in hospitals [35].
According to a systematic review of the literature studying the incidence of antibiotic resistance in West Africa, the resistance of *Staphylococcus aureus* to methicillin varied from one country to another, with a fairly high overall incidence (Table I) [48].

Table I. Frequency of *Staphylococcus aureus* resistance to meticillin in West African countries. Systematic review of the litterature, Africa, 2017.

Country	% resistance of *Staphylococcus aureus* to meticillin
Senegal and Niger	16
Nigeria	20 a 47
Benin	36

Togo	35.7
Ivory Coast	39

With regard to enterobacteria producing extended-spectrum b-lactamases (ESBL), their prevalence in these West African countries is considered very worrying. Taking *Eschirechia Coli* as an example, the proportion of ESBL-producing strains has reached 66% in Togo [48].

In Tunisia, a system for monitoring bacterial resistance in hospitals, AntibioResistance in Tunisia (LART), was set up in 1999. This was the first Tunisian network, the main objective of which is to monitor resistance to ATBs in the main bacterial species isolated in the main Tunisian university hospital centres, in order to follow the evolution of bacterial resistance and detect the emergence of new resistance phenotypes [49]. The evolution of resistance in the most frequently isolated species was studied and analysed each year. The latest results date back to 2017: - For *E. coli*, resistance to Amoxicillin and Ticarcillin reached more than 70% (Figure 15).

- *Klebsiella pneumoniae* resistance to Tetracycline exceeded 50% in 2017 (figure 16)
- For *S. aureus*, the most alarming percentage of resistance was to Penicillin and Amoxicillin, which has exceeded 90% since 2013 (figure 17).
- For *Pseudomonas aeruginosa* and *Acinetobacter baumanni*, resistance to Ticarcillin reached 20.2% and 86.1% respectively in 2017 (figure 18).

For Escherichia coli

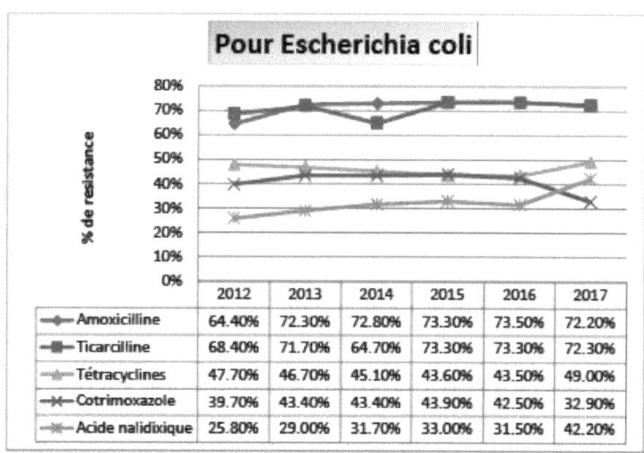

	2012	2013	2014	2015	2016	2017
Amoxicilline	64.40%	72.30%	72.80%	73.30%	73.50%	72.20%
Ticarcilline	68.40%	71.70%	64.70%	73.30%	73.30%	72.30%
Tétracyclines	47.70%	46.70%	45.10%	43.60%	43.50%	49.00%
Cotrimoxazole	39.70%	43.40%	43.40%	43.90%	42.50%	32.90%
Acide nalidixique	25.80%	29.00%	31.70%	33.00%	31.50%	42.20%

Figure 15. Evolution of the resistance of *'Escherichia coil* to different ATBs over the years. Data from LART (2012-2017)

For Klebsiella pneumoniae

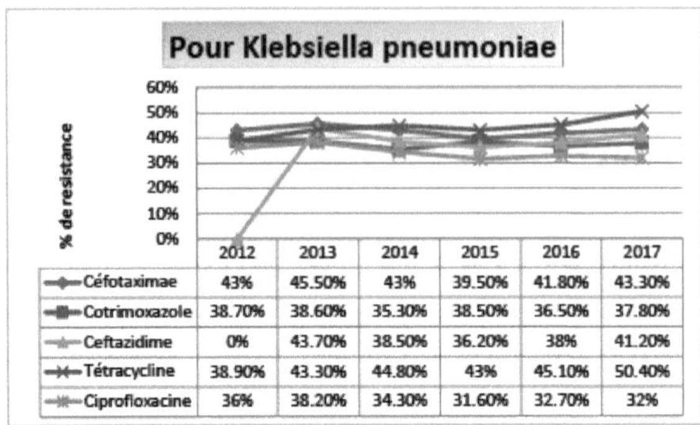

	2012	2013	2014	2015	2016	2017
Céfotaximae	43%	45.50%	43%	39.50%	41.80%	43.30%
Cotrimoxazole	38.70%	38.60%	35.30%	38.50%	36.50%	37.80%
Ceftazidime	0%	43.70%	38.50%	36.20%	38%	41.20%
Tétracycline	38.90%	43.30%	44.80%	43%	45.10%	50.40%
Ciprofloxacine	36%	38.20%	34.30%	31.60%	32.70%	32%

Figure 16. Trends in the resistance of *Klebsiella pneumoniae* to different ATBs over the years. Data from LART (2012-2017)

For Staphylococus aureus

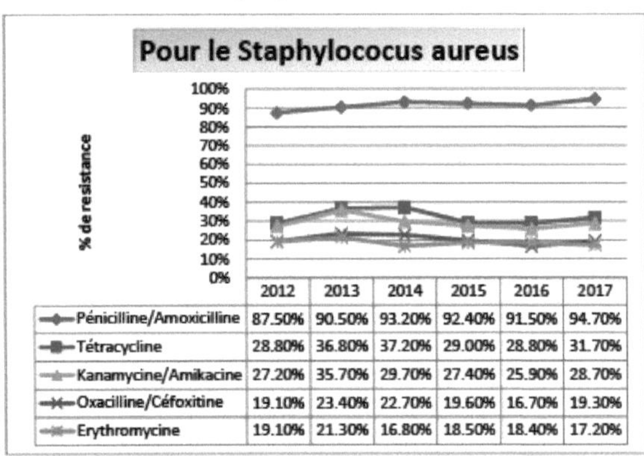

	2012	2013	2014	2015	2016	2017
Pénicilline/Amoxicilline	87.50%	90.50%	93.20%	92.40%	91.50%	94.70%
Tétracycline	28.80%	36.80%	37.20%	29.00%	28.80%	31.70%
Kanamycine/Amikacine	27.20%	35.70%	29.70%	27.40%	25.90%	28.70%
Oxacilline/Céfoxitine	19.10%	23.40%	22.70%	19.60%	16.70%	19.30%
Erythromycine	19.10%	21.30%	16.80%	18.50%	18.40%	17.20%

Figure 17. Trends in the resistance of *Staphylococcus aureus* to different ATBs over the years. Data from LART (2012-2017)

For Pseudomonas aeruginosa

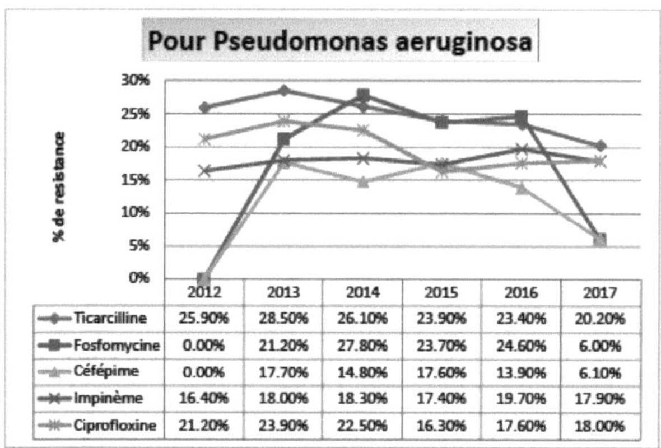

	2012	2013	2014	2015	2016	2017
Ticarcilline	25.90%	28.50%	26.10%	23.90%	23.40%	20.20%
Fosfomycine	0.00%	21.20%	27.80%	23.70%	24.60%	6.00%
Céfépime	0.00%	17.70%	14.80%	17.60%	13.90%	6.10%
Impinème	16.40%	18.00%	18.30%	17.40%	19.70%	17.90%
Ciprofloxine	21.20%	23.90%	22.50%	16.30%	17.60%	18.00%

Figure 18. Evolution of resistance in *Pseudomonas aeruginosa* to different ATBs over the years. Data from LART (2012-2017)

IV. Bibliographic synthesis

I.Bibliographical summary of the estimated impact of IAS

1.1 Methodology for calculating the impact of IAS

Incidence measures take into account the number of new cases of a disease observed during a given period, in a given place, in a given population.

They can therefore only be used when it is possible to distinguish, during a given period, between new cases and those which occurred before the start of the period.

There are two types of indicator: cumulative incidence (CI) and incidence density (ID):

1.1.1 Cumulative incidence (CI): calculated as follows:

number of new cases of HAIs

= in a population over a period T the total number of healthy people at risk at the start of the period T in question

Numerator: these are patients newly infected during the time period T

Denominator: this is the population at risk at the start of time period T.

The CI is a proportion and has no unit. It is expressed as x cases per 10^2 , 10^3 , 10^4 etc.

There are several scenarios for estimating the number of people at risk: If we consider that the composition of the groups studied is fixed at the start of the study and is not renewed during the study period, we speak of a closed or fixed cohort. There are several possible scenarios for estimating the number of people at risk:

- or the number of events, people lost to follow-up or deaths during the observation period is small compared with the initial population: the number of people at risk is then equal to P0, the population size at the start of the observation period.
- or this number is significant: the number of people at risk is then equal to

$$\frac{P0 + P1}{2}$$

With P1: population size at the end of the observation period.

1.1.2 Incidence density (ID)

It reflects the variation in the observation time for people at risk. It is useful for hospital monitoring, and is calculated as follows:

$$DI = \frac{\substack{\text{nombre de nouveaux cas survenus des IAS} \\ \text{dans une population pendant une période T}}}{\substack{\text{somme des personnes−temps} \\ \text{pendant la même periode de temps T}}} \text{ X 100}$$

number of new cases of HAIs

in a population during a period T

sum of person-time

during the same period T

Numerator: these are patients newly infected during the time period T

Denominator: this is the total length of hospitalisation for patients at risk (in days).
This measure should be used when the period during which the incidence of an event can be studied (during population monitoring) varies from one subject to another.
It is expressed in person-time at risk (time: months or years).
It measures the speed at which a disease spreads.
For an unstable population such as the hospital population, there are many arrivals and departures (discharges, transfers, deaths, etc.) and many people are lost to view.
So not all patients have the same length of exposure for the same length of time.
It is therefore more accurate than CI, especially when the proportion of people lost to follow-up is high in a study population.
For example: an incidence density of 10/100,000 person-years means that there were 10 new cases of infection for every 100,000 people monitored over the course of a year.

Principle of the PERSON-TIME concept

- Each subject is no longer counted for the whole of the observation period planned for the entire population, but only for the period during which it was possible to observe this subject, before the occurrence of the event under study. This period is referred to as the risk period.

The total number of person-time for a given population is equal to the sum of the follow-up carried out by all the subjects in this population in number of person-time.

- The benefits of impact surveys :

Longitudinal studies provide information on the spread of HCAIs.
The main advantages of impact surveys are :

- Objectivise the risk of infection: i.e. the probability of a HAI occurring in the future
- Identify the risk factors for these HCAIs
- Optimal approach to the cost of these infections

The results obtained from this type of survey are characterised by their reliability and accuracy. For a population of hospitalised patients, incidence measurement remains the better indicator of the risk of acquiring a HCAI than prevalence measurement [50].

- The disadvantages of incidence surveys :

Incidence surveys also have a number of drawbacks:

- The cost of this type of study is high, as it requires staff trained in the data collection method and greater logistical resources.
- This type of survey may require data to be collected over a longer period, resulting in a heavier workload.

1.2 Discussion of literature findings

A multicentre (2010-2015) surveillance survey of medical device-associated infections (MDSI) conducted by the International Nosocomial Infection Control Consortium

(INICC) in 50 countries on different continents (in Latin America, Europe, the Eastern Mediterranean, South-East Asia and the Western Pacific), in medical and surgical intensive care units, found an incidence density of CVC-related bacteremia equal to 4.2 per 1000 CVC days. Comparing these results with those reported by the National Health-care Safety Network (NHSN) in 2012 in the United States, this ID was almost 5 times higher. The ID for pneumonia associated with mechanical ventilation (PAVM) was also higher (13 versus 0.9 infections per 1000 ventilation days) as was the ID for urinary tract infections (UTI) associated with urinary catheterisation (5 versus 1.7 per 1000 catheterisation days) [51].

These variations in the results observed in these two studies could be explained by the lack of compliance with guidelines, the low nurse/patient ratio, the lack of training and experience of paramedical staff, the overcrowding and overloading of hospitals and the lack of medical supplies [51].

A randomised controlled trial of HAIs in intensive care units in one European country, the Republic of Cyprus, showed that the overall CI of HAIs was 12.6% and the DI was 19 HAIs per 1000 days of intensive care. Infections due to CVCs were the most frequent, with a cumulative incidence of almost 50%, followed by VAPs (37%) and UTIs related to urinary catheterisation (14%) [52].

In fact, the risk of infection in intensive care units (ICUs) is particularly greater than for patients in conventional hospital settings [53,54]. These high figures in intensive care settings are generally related to the severity of underlying co-morbidities, the relatively fragile condition of these patients, the multiplicity of therapies prescribed, and the almost systematic and frequent use of various DM [51,55].

Another prospective multicentre study conducted in 2019 by the INICC in intensive care units in 42 countries with limited resources, focusing on CVP-related bacteremia, found an incidence density of 2.4/1000 CVP per day with a mortality rate attributable to the infection of 18% [56]. This result was similar to that observed in another multicentre study, with a similar methodology, conducted by the INICC in the Middle East in 2013 (ID of 2.3 per 1000 *VSC* per day). However, the mortality observed in this study was much higher (29% versus 18%) [57].

Although studies are rare in developing countries, according to the WHO, the morbidity of these infections in these countries is significantly higher than in developed countries [58].

A survey of the incidence of HCAIs in South Africa showed that the incidence density of HCAIs exceeded 30 cases per 1000 patient days in hospital [59]. Comparable results were reported by a longitudinal study conducted in Ethiopia in 2016, with an overall ID of 28 cases per 1000 person-days. This ID was 4 times higher in ICUs than in other wards, exceeding 207 cases per 1000 patient-days [38].

These results were higher than those found by the INICC in Morocco, with an ID of 22 HCAIs per 1000 hospital days, with a predominance of VAPs, with a density of 43 per 1000 ventilator days [60]. The impact of HAIs is particularly felt in countries with poor human and material resources, given the shortage of healthcare staff and the absence of prevention strategies aimed at compliance with preliminary hygiene

measures, and the absence of regulations relating to the mandatory reporting and monitoring of these infections in healthcare establishments [61].
This phenomenon is increasingly exacerbated in countries with limited resources by the low level of spending on combating these infections on the one hand, and by the emergence of antimicrobial resistance on the other [8].
Furthermore, the disparity in results observed between different countries, and even within the same country (from one department to another), can be explained by several factors. There are factors that depend on the characteristics of the patients and the heterogeneity of the intrinsic and extrinsic risk of the population studied, and other factors that are linked to the variations and methodological differences adopted, such as: the type of prospective or retrospective study, the data collection method, the differences in the definitions of the infections used and the variations in the methodologies for calculating the indicators used.
The comparison must also take into account whether or not there is an effective programme to combat infectious diseases and the level of control of infectious risk at hospital and ward level.
Between 1995 and 2010, the WHO reported a morbidity rate of IN of almost 18% in Morocco and Tunisia [58]. It also highlighted the scarcity of available data in all low- and middle-income countries, which leads to a real under- or over-estimation of these infections [13].
Tunisia, a developing country with limited human and material resources, is affected by this problem, but studies determining its scale and consequences are limited [62].
According to a Tunisian survey conducted in the intensive care unit of Kairouan [63] in 2014, studying the incidence of UTIs and their risk factors, the overall incidence exceeded 30% with an ID reaching 55 UTIs per 1000 days of hospitalisation. VAPs were the most dominant, followed by UTIs related to bladder catheterisation and CVC bacteremia, with respectively IDs of 54.8, 12 and 11.2 per 1000 days of corresponding DM.
Comparing these results with other studies of incidence in intensive care settings [61,64] conducted at national level, we note differences, but these figures are considered to be high overall.
Among these studies, one was conducted in 2012 in a Tunisian intensive care unit in Sousse, focusing on the incidence of HAIs [61]. The overall incidence of these infections was 16.2%, with an ID of 17 infected patients per 1000 days of hospitalisation. CVC-related infections were the most frequent, followed by CVP-related infections.
The ID of CVC-related infections was twice that observed in Colombia [65] and seven times higher than that reported in the United States [66]. The choice of CVC insertion site and compliance with aseptic measures and standard hygiene precautions during insertion, maintenance, handling and removal of this type of catheter are the main determining factors in reducing the associated risk of infection [22,23,61].
Similarly, CVPs are a major source of hospital-acquired infections. They are among

the most commonly used medical devices in healthcare establishments worldwide. As reported in an international multicentre study conducted in 42 countries worldwide, approximately 200 million CVPs are inserted into healthcare facilities each year in the United States, with an ICU ID of CVP-related infections of 2.4 per 1000 CVP days [56].

A Tunisian study conducted in 2017, looking at the incidence of adverse events related to VCTs (AE-VCTs) in a cardiology department, found an overall incidence of AE-VCTs of over 30%. Infections accounted for 11.4% of all recorded AEs [67].

The high incidence of vascular catheter-related infections is due to a lack of compliance with standard hygiene rules, and to the absence of programmes for monitoring and reporting this type of infection in health facilities.

Infections related to vascular devices (CVCs and CVPs) are generally the consequence of the quality of insertion, maintenance care, the time taken to remove the device and the length of stay [68]. They depend on several factors: the patient's condition, the place of hospitalisation, the type of equipment used, the products and treatments infused, the insertion site, hygiene measures, the length of time the venous line is maintained and the diagnostic criterion chosen, etc[61,69] ▪

Furthermore, surgical site infections (SSI) are considered to be among the most frequent complications in patients undergoing surgical procedures, constituting a major source of morbidity and mortality in these patients. According to a prospective study aimed at estimating the incidence of SSI after caesarean section in a maternity ward in the region of Kairouan in 2015, the overall incidence was 5% with an ID of 1.7 per 1000 patient-days [70].

These results were similar to those observed in the United States. However, these figures were higher in Niger and India (reaching 24%) [70].

This type of maternal infection is much higher in developing countries (incidence of up to 27%) than in developed countries (incidence of 7%) [71,72].

The majority of SSIs are due to bacterial inoculations during incisions. These infections can be prevented by practising a set of best clinical practices (BCPs) that minimise the development of these infections [73].

Preparation for surgery should always include a shower bath, appropriate administration of surgical antibiotic prophylaxis (selecting the right ATB with a dose adapted to the patient's weight and administration at the right time before the surgical procedure and not exceeding 24 hours) and good cutaneous asepsis of the surgical site [73,74].

2. Summary of the literature on estimating the additional costs associated with IAS

2.1 The different methods for calculating the additional cost of a project
to IAS

The medico-economic impact of HCAIs continues to grow worldwide.

A better assessment of the costs associated with HCAIs could mobilise decision-makers to improve the quality of the care offered and limit the rise in these expenses through financial investment in the development of relevant prevention and surveillance strategies.

2.1.1 The different types of IAS costs :

Table II. Different types of IAS-related costs.

Hospital costs	Known in particular as summary costs, they are represented by : -directly invoiced medical costs such as: additional radiological and bacteriological tests, therapeutic treatment, etc. -Unbilled medical costs corresponding to the additional workload and included in the price of a day's hospitalisation.
Post-hospital costs invoices	These are all the costs corresponding to follow-up treatment, outpatient care, loss of productivity and convalescence time.
Prevention costs	Are represented by the effectiveness of the prevention measures put in place in a given healthcare establishment

2.1.2 Cost estimation methods

Various calculation methods are available to help assess the additional costs associated with IAS. There are :

> Direct estimation :

This is also known as the "accounting" method. It consists of measuring the additional costs (medication, tests, length of stay, etc.) for each infected patient.

Chaix et al used this method in a French survey. They obtained an estimated extra cost of $9275, equivalent to £8483.84 ($1 = £0.91) [75].

> Estimated by the doctor:

This is a method whereby a clinical expert subjectively estimates whether the cause of death in patients is due to one or more HCAIs or not. He or she then records the exact additional costs of ancillary services (bacteriological tests, X-rays, antibiotics, etc.) as well as the specific routine costs for each infected patient. These are then compared with the hospital bill using a cost analyst. [76]

According to Haley RW, this method underestimates the real value of costs, since these expenses are calculated only if they were clearly the result of an IAS [77].

> Case-control comparison :

This method consists of measuring the cost of treating a subgroup of infected patients, then comparing it with the cost of treating a subgroup of non-infected patients with the same characteristics (sex, associated pathologies, age, treatment, etc.) to ensure the objectivity of the results [75].

According to some authors, this method can have disadvantages such as :

- non-comparability of groups
- the insufficient number of witnesses chosen

> Simple comparison :

This method involves comparing the additional costs incurred by a group of infected patients with the costs incurred by a group of non-infected patients, who do not necessarily have the same characteristics.

This method may not be satisfactory, as the groups selected may differ, particularly in terms of the underlying pathologies, which could lead to an overestimation of costs.

2.2 Choice of method :

The choice of method for estimating additional hospital costs varies according to the data available. In fact, these factors depend on several parameters such as :

- Resources provided to carry out the survey
- the quality of medical records
- the option of computerised data processing...

2.3 Economic analysis :

According to the literature on the economic analysis of additional costs attributed to IAS, two types of model are valid:

> Cost-benefit analysis :

The aim of this approach is to express in real budgetary terms the benefits of applying preventive procedures to significantly reduce the additional costs associated with IAS.

If the cost of HCAI is less than the cost of the preventive measures taken, they should be replaced by other, more advantageous and less costly measures. Conversely, if these actions are beneficial in terms of financial gain, they should be monitored and adopted in order to develop appropriate systems for compliance and control of effective preventive measures [78].

> Cost-effectiveness analysis :

This approach aims to express costs in terms of quality. In other words, it will make it possible to explain expenditure in terms of survival and morbidity, where a cost/effectiveness ratio can be assigned.

2.4 Discussion of the results of the literature :

According to the WHO, the annual cost of infections contracted in the course of care in the UK is estimated at £1 billion. In the United States of America, the annual cost is estimated at between 4.5 and 5.7 billion dollars. In Mexico, the annual cost is almost 1.5 billion dollars [9].

The results found in the literature have demonstrated a significant relationship between longer hospital stays and the additional costs attributed to them.

According to a study carried out in a Thai hospital in 2013, the acquisition of one or more INs was responsible for an 8.75 ± 1.28 day extension of the duration of hospitalisation, generating additional costs of $2.50993 ± 979.74 [79].

The authors also evaluated the cost of the additional stay for each type of infection, highlighting the increased expenditure due to CVC-related bacteremia, as shown in the following table (table III):

Table III. Cost and length of stay attributable to each type of infection,

Thailand, 2013

	Cost ($)	Length of stay
CVC-related bacteria	2.50993	24.94
UTI related to urinary catheterisation	1.05454	5.83
Infection of tract lower respiratory	1.89317	6.06

The occurrence of NI is likely to lead to complications in patients, resulting in a longer duration of treatment and significantly higher expenditure.

In the same study, the authors assessed the effectiveness of implementing a new strategy for the application of measures to combat IN. The aim of these measures was to increase the number of preventive measures by combining them with monitoring and control of infected patients by specialised teams, thereby minimising or eliminating the risk factors that encourage the acquisition of nosocomial infections. They demonstrated the effectiveness of these new measures, which were less costly and saved $20,444.62 [79].

Similarly, according to another study carried out in two paediatric and neonatal wards in Greece, CVC-related bacteremia was responsible for a considerable prolongation of the stay of 21 days and an additional cost of £13,727 [80].

They demonstrated a significant difference in the additional length of stay and associated extra costs between patients with CVC bacteremia and those without, as shown below:

Table IV. Prolonged costs and durations due to HCAIs using a linear regression model

	Infected patients	Non-infected patients
Additional length of stay (in days)		
Costs (£)	131.302	17.788

The methods used in this study to estimate direct medical costs were based on an approach that calculates micro-costs. These data were collected by referring to patient records, then combined with unit costs of care expressed in Euros:

- The extra costs of additional examinations: have been obtained from the official website of the Greek public health insurance fund "E.O.P.Y.Y".
- The costs of medical supplies used to manage the CVCs were obtained from the Observe Net website, which provides unit costs for public hospitals, and then multiplied by the number of services provided.
- Surgical costs: were obtained from the surgical costs of private hospitals using the direct estimation method. Profits were deducted from the cost of each operation.

^ In conclusion, the additional costs associated with HCAI were calculated by combining the costs associated with extending the length of stay with the daily cost.

- Additional costs due to medication (ATB, ATV...), are equal to :

Daily dose of each drug * Number of days of drug use * Unit price of drugs in (mg/ml...).

This cost has been calculated on the basis of the unit prices established by the factories after application of the necessary provisions for discounts and rebates.

In most studies, the direct financial additional cost is the most calculated. This leads to a poor estimate of the exact cost of the infection, and there may therefore be an overestimate or underestimate of the real cost of hospital-acquired infections. These direct additional costs are generally due to an increase in the consumption of healthcare, longer hospital stays and increased consumption of anti-infectious agents for diagnosis and treatment. These factors explain most of the direct additional financial costs caused by HCAIs [81].

According to a study evaluating the impact of nosocomial infections on paediatric hospitalisation costs in Sao Paulo, Brazil, estimated expenditure on patients with nosocomial infections was 4 times higher than on non-infected patients. This was due to an extended stay of 14 days. They used the following method to calculate the additional costs [26] :

The individual calculation of costs for each child was estimated by multiplying the number of days of hospitalisation by the daily hospitalisation costs corresponding to the month and sector of hospitalisation.

This extremely high cost in infected patients ($39,66821) may be due to the presence of more than one infection or complication caused by IN as well as exposure to invasive procedures [26].

In addition, hospital-acquired infections are becoming a growing cause for concern, given the increasing frequency of antibiotic resistance in hospitals. In this same study, the authors estimated the additional cost due to antibiotic resistance by calculating the unit dose of each ATB for each patient throughout the treatment period, without including costs due to losses such as contamination of bottles, breakage, etc.

As a result, they found that patients who received treatment for an infection were almost 4 times more expensive than those who did not.

This increase may be justified by the need to use new, more effective types of TBA with a broader spectrum of activity, which may be more expensive than conventional treatments [26].

The longer hospital stays observed may be explained by the lack of diagnostic procedures for early detection of these infections.

According to a study carried out in South Africa in 2015, HAIs resulted in an additional stay of 2275 days, responsible for additional costs of 371887$ [59].

To estimate this burden, they calculated the extra cost by multiplying the number of events per HCAI site by the median excess length of stay for that site and then by the unit cost per day (including laboratory, radiology and pharmacy costs, etc.).

However, 95% of IN events required new antimicrobial treatment, resulting in 2365 days of hospitalization and an additional cost of $14,730 [59].

In the same vein, the HASSAN II University Hospital in Morocco has published the results of a study carried out in 2011, aimed at estimating the additional expenditure due to hospital-acquired infections in the following three departments: intensive care, surgery and medicine.

These costs were of the order of 1165922.05 DH, with an additional cost related to the additional stay of 72900 DH. They also estimated an annual cost related to these infections of 15008628.96 DH, with a large share going to intensive care units [10] (Figure 19).

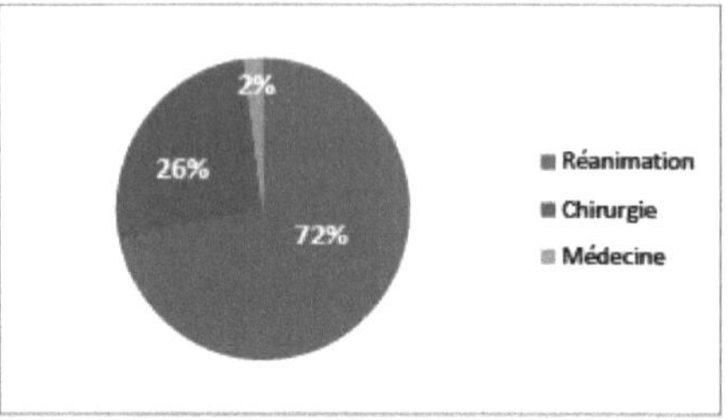

- Resuscitation
- Surgery
- Medicine

Figure 19. Breakdown of annual expenditure related to the treatment of IN by department. Survey CHU HASSAN II, Morocco, 2011

They also estimated a prevention cost of around DH6,8800. In order to estimate the annual expenditure lost, they used the following methods of calculation:

- Cost of infection = Cost of general expenses + Cost of additional examinations + Cost of antibiotic treatment
- Unit cost of prevention = cost of each basic means of prevention used by medical and paramedical staff (clean, sterile gloves, bleach, detergents, disposable paper, washbasins, liquid soap, etc.).
- Overall cost of prevention = unit cost of each means of prevention* number of patients
- Additional costs = costs of infection - costs of prevention
- Annual cost = additional costs *prevalence of new infections

An evaluation study of the additional cost of IN at the Tizi Ouzou University Hospital in Algeria estimated the additional cost of hospitalisation to be 6,801,953.40 DA, and the cost of prevention to be 12 times lower [82].

To approximate this expenditure, the authors estimated the additional cost for each infected patient of prolonged hospitalisation due to NI.

Studies determining the extra cost of HCAI are rare in Tunisia. According to an old study carried out at the HCN in Tunis in 1998 on the incidence of HCAI and the approach to their extra cost, the extra length of stay estimated by simple comparison between the infected group and the non-infected group was 9.3 days. The extra cost attributed to IN was 20,496 DT for the cost related to length of stay and 4302.707 DT for the cost related to ATBs [50].

These results are probably inferior to the reality because the calculation of additional costs was based on the fixed price per day of hospitalisation, without taking into account in detail the costs of diagnostic examinations and care provided [50].

The results of studies estimating the additional costs of hospital-acquired infections differ and vary for several reasons. The type of hospital, the department chosen, the calculation method, the size of the target population and the sites of infection studied are all factors that lead to heterogeneity in these results.

V. Measures to combat HCAIs

Combating HCAIs is a vital step in ensuring patient safety and improving the quality of care.

Standard precautions are considered to be the cornerstone of all prevention of person-to-person transmission, applicable in all situations.

Their overriding principle is to consider every patient as a potential carrier of a known or unknown infectious agent.

Their purpose is to protect staff and patients.

Standard precautions must be applied by all healthcare professionals to all patients. They essentially comprise :

1. Hand hygiene

It is recognised worldwide as the key to preventing NI. Its effectiveness has been widely demonstrated. The aim of this measure is to reduce the risk of infection by limiting hand-held transmission. The contaminated hands of healthcare staff represent a potential source of transmission of pathogenic agents in healthcare establishments. Patients can become colonised or infected through contact with colonised staff. Staff can be decolonised if hand hygiene is respected (Figure 20).

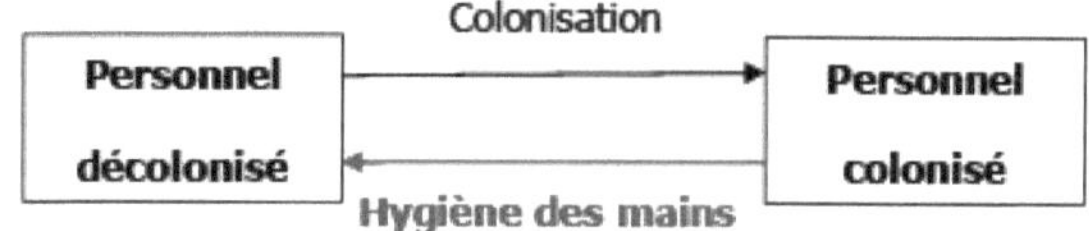

Colonisation

Decolonised staff Colonised staff

Hand hygiene

Figure 20: Diagram illustrating the importance of hand hygiene

Since 2005, the WHO has taken the initiative and been involved in developing a programme to promote "Clean Care is Safer Care" hand hygiene [83].

It published the first version of a set of hand hygiene guidelines in 2006 and the final version in 2009, which highlighted a multimodal strategy to improve hand hygiene practice [83].

The commitment of healthcare staff in the fight against the transmission of infectious diseases is a decisive factor in reducing this risk. This can be achieved by applying and complying with simple hygiene gestures and rules.

The WHO recommends that healthcare staff wash their hands frequently with soap and water or with a hydroalcoholic solution. According to the WHO, there are 5 essential indications or times when staff should wash their hands during medical care [84]: (figure 21)

1- Before patient contact
2- Before the aseptic procedure (e.g. insertion of devices such as catheters)
3- After the risk of exposure to a biological fluid
4- After contact with the patient
5- After contact with the patient's environment

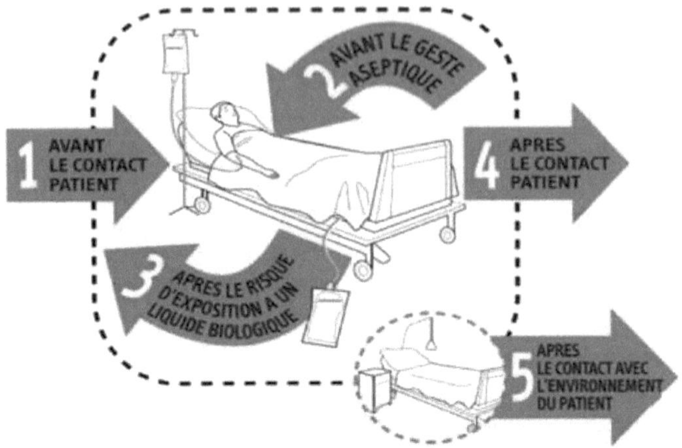

Figure 21: The 5 key moments in hand washing recommended by the WHO

1.1 Types of hand washing

There are different types of hand washing, which differ in terms of duration and the act that follows (table V):

Table V. Different types of hand washing

Techniques	Simple wash	Antiseptic washing	Surgical washing	Disinfection
Objectives	Reduce the number of micro-organisms			
	Removing scales and dirt			
			Reducing resident flora	
Product	Mild liquid soap in a dispenser, not including antiseptic	Broad-spectrum antiseptic soap in dispenser	Product bactericide	Hydro-alcoholic solution
Duration	30 seconds	1 minute	5 minutes	30 seconds

1.2 Simple hand washing steps

The hand washing steps are illustrated as follows: (Figure 22)

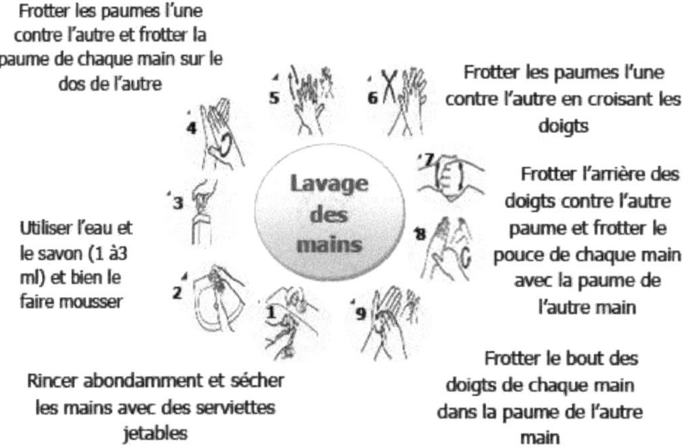

Rub palms together and the palm of each hand against the back of the other.
Rub palms together, crossing fingers
Rub the back of the fingers against the other palm and rub the thumb of each hand with the palm of the other hand Rub the fingertips of each hand in the palm of the other hand
Use water and soap (1 to 3 ml) and lather well.
Rinse hands thoroughly and dry with disposable towels

Figure 22. Stages of simple hand washing

According to the literature, it has been widely demonstrated that interventions focusing on the promotion of and compliance with hand hygiene rules are an effective means of limiting the frequency of the occurrence of nosocomial infections and the associated additional costs. Gagne et al concluded after a cost-benefit analysis that the practice of and compliance with hand hygiene saved $688,843 per hospitalisation [85].

Pokrywka et al. carried out an intervention in 2014 in the USA, aimed at reducing *Clostridium Difcie* infection (CDI) in a 520-bed hospital. This intervention consisted of distributing educational leaflets, reminder signs and alcohol-based wipes on meal trays, and involving staff in helping patients clean their hands at mealtimes, which contributed to a reduction in the rate of CDI from 10.5 per 10,000 patient days to 7 per 10,000 patient days over one year [86].

Other authors in Canada studied the impact of raising patient and visitor awareness of the importance of hand hygiene, distributing brochures on HCAIs and cleaning patients' hands with a disinfectant twice a day. They found a reduction of almost half in the rate of HCAIs due to *methiciiiin-resistant Staphyiococcus* (from 10.6 per 1000 admissions before the intervention to 5.2 per 1000 admissions after the intervention) and a 30% increase in workers' compliance with hand hygiene (table VI) [85].

Table VI. Summary of different interventional studies on hand hygiene

Authors	Elementsof intervention	Results
Pokrywka et al [86] (2014)	Education, recall signals, product supply	The DCI rate fell from 10.5 per 10,000 patient days to 7 per 10,000 patient days.
Gagne et al [85] (2010)	Education, supply product	-MRSA rate halved. -Increasing hand hygiene compliance among healthcare workers.
Ardizzane et al [87] (2013)	Training for healthcare staff	-27% increase in the overall proportion of workers helping with hand hygiene
Arntz et al (2016) Jeans et al (2017)	Education, monitoring, reminders, comments	-increase in hand hygiene compliance among healthcare staff: to 46% and 92% respectively

2. Sterilisation and disinfection of medical equipment

2.1 Sterilisation

Sterilisation is an essential element in the fight against infectious diseases. It enables patients to receive care with medical and surgical equipment that is free of all micro-organisms. It applies to heat-stable medical and surgical instruments and linen.

There are different methods of sterilisation:

> *Steam sterilisation*

It is considered the reference technique, used for all thermostable medical devices.

- Advantages
- Best heat transfer agent
- Effective against non-conventional transmissible agents
- No toxic residues
- Low cost

> *Sterilisation with dry lime*

This technique is performed in a Poupinel oven. Its use is limited to materials sensitive to water vapour.

This type has a number of drawbacks and should no longer be used: - Air is a poor conductor of heat - The load must be correctly positioned - Possible oxidation of metal objects - Alteration of sharp instruments - Does not sterilise textiles.

> *Gas sterilisation (ethylene oxide and formaldehyde)*

> *Sterilisation by ionising radiation*

The best sterilisation method for any object is one that reliably destroys all micro-organisms and/or spores without damaging the object.

2.2 Disinfection

This is a momentary operation that eliminates or kills micro-organisms and/or inactivates undesirable viruses carried by contaminated inert media. It is used for heat-sensitive materials.

Transmission of HAI by contaminated equipment is often suspected in hospitals. There is a precise disinfection protocol describing the appropriate procedure for each type of medical device (table VII).

Table VII. Classification of medical and treatment devices required.

	Non critical	Non-sterilisable critical and semi-critical	Sterilisable critical and semi-critical
	In contact with healthy skin: tourniquet, Kocher forceps, tray, tensiometer. stethoscope...	In contact with non-invasive mucosa or non-intact skin: mask, insufflator. bronchial and digestive endoscope...	Medio-surgical instrumentation, joint endoscope, ccel ioscope...
Procedure	P1	P2	P3
Stage 1	Pre-desinfection Ringage	Pre-desinfection Ringage	Pre-desinfection Ringage
Stage 2	Cleaning Ringage Drying Manual tomatises	Cleaning Ringage drying Manual tomatises	Cleaning Ringage Drying Manual"au tomatises
Step 3	Clean use	Disinfection by immersion Ringage drying	Sterilisation by autoclaving
Equipment	OWN	DESINFECTE	STERILE
	Storage	Storage	Storage
		Immediate use or deferred use (after ncc/.vMk? d^sirfecticnl	

3. Rational use of antibiotics

Controlling antibiotic therapy within a healthcare establishment requires the implementation of an ATB policy in the hospital with the aim of restricting their use. Prophylactic antibiotic therapy is only permitted in the preoperative phase, for a maximum of 24 hours, and for the prevention of infections caused by gas-forming anaerobes in traumatology.

Φ Proper use of ATBs considerably reduces the occurrence of HAIs.

Emine Alp et al have proposed a strategy for preventing the emergence of resistant bacteria in intensive care settings, based on five main measures [89] :

1. Implementation of HCAI control and prevention measures, and isolation of infected patients to avoid cross-infection.
2. Early detection of infections based on effective HCAI surveillance and treatment strategies.
3. Rational use of broad-spectrum ATBs and prophylactic ATBs before surgery.
4. Training and education of staff in the correct use of antimicrobials.
5. Implementation of plans for monitoring the use of ATBs in accordance with the guidelines.

Other additional measures may be adopted, such as adapting guidelines for prescribing ATBs, and producing annual reports providing data on the most prevalent micro-organisms in health facilities.

Tunisia has committed to implementing a national plan to combat the spread of resistant bacteria for 2019-2023, with four main objectives [49] :

- Increase awareness and understanding of the problem of antimicrobial resistance through effective communication, education and training.

- Strengthen knowledge and the evidence base through surveillance and research.
- Reduce the incidence of infections through effective sanitation, hygiene and infection prevention measures.
- Optimising the use of antimicrobial drugs in human and animal health

4. Other preventive measures

4.1 Isolation

The aim of isolation measures is to prevent the circulation of germs by creating barriers that prevent all forms of possible contact between patients and sources of colonisation [14].

Isolation combines geographical and technical measures. There are 2 types of isolation [90] :

- Septic isolation: aims to control the spread of germs from a colonised or infected patient. It involves isolating a patient with a bacterial or viral infection, or a patient colonised by a germ, who poses a risk to other patients or staff.

Precautions are taken on discharge to protect the environment and other patients.

- Protective isolation: Patients sometimes require isolation because of their increased susceptibility to infection. This type of isolation is used to protect a patient at high risk of infection (fragile or immunocompromised) from the hospital environment, other patients or even visitors.

Precautions are particularly important when *entering* the room to protect the infected patient.

NB: isolation measures are no longer effective unless hands are washed between each treatment.

A study carried out in respiratory intensive care units demonstrated the role of isolation rooms in reducing nosocomial infections by minimising the risk of cross-transmission [91].

4.2 Training for care staff

Training healthcare staff and raising their awareness of hospital hygiene is an essential part of preventing hospital-acquired infections. It must be specific and adapted to the needs of each healthcare establishment. It requires consensus and the motivation and support of all hospital staff. Hygiene training and education is ideally offered to all hospital departments and all healthcare staff, with priority given to high-risk infection departments such as intensive care, surgery and neonatology [14].

4.3 Business attire

Contact with professional clothing can cause contamination. Germs living on the surface of coats can, with the accumulation over time of various types of soiling, find a climate of nourishment favourable to their development. It is therefore essential to prevent transmission via clothing. Clothing must be appropriate for the activity being carried out.

- Gowns should be changed daily and whenever they become soiled [92].
- Goggles and masks must be worn for high-risk treatments [93].

- the wearing of a cap and shoes or boots is sometimes necessary, especially in high-risk departments [93].

4.4 Wearing gloves

Gloves must be changed between two patients or two activities (including for the same patient). They should be put on just before contact, care or treatment, and removed at the end of care and discarded before touching the environment [92.93].

5. Infection prevention by infection site

5.1 CVC-related bacteria

Bacterial infections due to vascular catheterisation represent a major risk. There is a high mortality rate, and survivors only recover at the cost of a very significant increase in the length of hospital stay [50].

The financial cost of these infections is therefore considerable [94]. Preventive measures aimed at reducing this risk, such as those proposed by the CDC [94], include the following, depending on the stage of the invasive procedure:

- Before and during insertion

o If possible, avoid the femoral vein for central venous catheter insertion.

o Use sterile precautionary barriers.

o Prepare the skin with Chlorhexidine.

o Apply a dressing impregnated with Chlorhexidine.

- After insertion

o Bathe patients in intensive care units daily with Chlorhexidine.

o Rapidly remove non-essential intravascular catheters

5.2 Urinary tract infections associated with urinary catheterisation

To prevent these infections, it is best to :

- Insert a urinary catheter only if necessary
- Position the probe only for as long as necessary
- Maintain a firm, unobstructed drainage system below the level of the bladder at all times.

5.3 Pneumopathies associated with mechanical ventilation

A prevention policy could reduce the frequency of these infections, as well as the morbidity and secondary mortality associated with them. It is preferable to :

- Promoting non-invasive positive pressure ventilation.
- Keep mechanically ventilated patients in a semi-recumbent position rather than supine.
- Regular antiseptic oral care.

5.4 Surgical site infection [95]

- Remove hair before the operation only if necessary, using clippers rather than razors.
- Check glucose levels adequately before the operation.
- Pre-operative prophylactic antibiotics targeted at the most common pathogens,

not to exceed 24 hours post-operatively.

- Treating infections away from the surgical site before elective surgery (optional)

VI. drawing up a survey protocol and questionnaire

1. Study protocol: Estimation of the incidence and approach to the additional cost of nosocomial infections in surgical and intensive care settings at the HCN in Tunis.

1.1 Introduction (Justification for the study)

HAIs are now a global public health priority. They are considered to be the most undesirable and frequent event in healthcare delivery threatening patient safety worldwide [37].

They represent a major health and economic burden, with considerable morbidity and mortality among hospitalised patients [8,96,97,98].

This problem is even more frequent and more serious in developing countries [2]. However, according to the WHO, few studies and publications have been carried out on this subject [99], which means that the extent of the burden in these countries is underestimated [13].

Tunisia has not been spared this scourge, with a national prevalence of HAIs estimated at 7.7% [12] and exceeding 25% in medical intensive care units [13]. Indeed, ICUs are considered to be the epicentre and main source of emerging problems of HAIs and antimicrobial resistance in hospitals [100]. This is due to the frequent use of invasive procedures and multiple therapeutic prescriptions, as well as the fragile nature of these patients [101].

Similarly, SSI in the surgical setting represents a major burden in terms of patient morbidity and mortality and additional costs [102,103].

According to the latest survey of the prevalence of hospital-acquired infections at the HCN in Tunis, adult medical ICUs and surgical hospitalization units were among the hospitalization sectors with the highest prevalence of infections, at 30.8% and 12.1% respectively.

However, a significant proportion of SSIs, and NIs in general, can be prevented by effective surveillance and control programmes [102].

In fact, epidemiological surveillance is the first fundamental step towards controlling and preventing these infections [14,15].

Incidence surveys are the gold standard for monitoring hospital-acquired infections. They provide a precise and rigorous estimate of the risk of nosocomial infection in healthcare establishments [14].

In addition, nosocomial infections impose a heavy financial burden on healthcare systems [27]. It is therefore necessary to study the economic impact of these infections. This will make it possible to quantify the scale of the expenditure and consequent financial loss to hospitals. This will provide quantified evidence to convince decision-makers of the importance of investing in preventive measures and in the fight against these infections, given the considerable gains that can be achieved in return [34].

In Tunisia, there is a lack of precise, up-to-date analysis of the epidemiological situation with regard to nosocomial infections, with essentially a paucity of data concerning the estimated incidence and attributable cost of these infections.

This subject is under-researched, particularly in intensive care and surgical settings. Hence the need for this type of study to guide and better target prevention programmes against nosocomial infections and to improve and adapt surveillance and control practices.
In order to make up for the lack of data and studies in this context in our health establishment (HCN), we aim with this study to :

- Determining the incidence of INFECTIONS in the surgical and intensive care environment at the HCN of Tunis.
- To estimate the additional medical cost of these infections, represented by the increased length of stay and consumption of antibiotics.

1.2 Methodology

1.2.1 Type of survey

This is a descriptive observational study, of the cohort type (incidence study) with prospective (longitudinal) data collection, which will be spread over 3 months and will be carried out in the general surgery departments A and B and the anaesthesia and intensive care department of the HCN in Tunis.

1.2.2 Survey population

- **Inclusion criteria**

All patients newly admitted to the survey department (who will be hospitalised from midnight on the day the survey begins) and who are healthy (free of IN on admission) and who have been in hospital for more than 48 hours (>=48H) will be included.

- **Non-inclusion criteria**

Our survey will not include :

- Former patients of the department (hospitalised before the start of our survey)
- Patients transferred from another HCN establishment or department (whether infected or not).

1.2.3 Investigation tool and data to be collected

Information will be collected using a questionnaire form for each patient.
This sheet will consist of two parts:
> A section common to all patients containing: o General information about the patient o Reason for hospitalisation
o Intrinsic risk factors:

- Mac CABE gravity score
- Medical history (diabetes, hypertension, chronic respiratory insufficiency, smoking, alcohol, etc.)
- Terrain: immunodepression, progressive neoplasia.

o Extrinsic risk factors: Invasive devices and procedures (CVP, CVC, urinary catheter, intubation, mechanical ventilation, gastric tube, etc.).
o Surgical variables: surgical route, type of surgery, nature of anaesthesia, ASA score, NNIS score, antibiotic prophylaxis.

o Initial infectious state of the patient

> Another section devoted to patients with one or more infections: information on the date of diagnosis of the infection, the site of infection, the samples taken, the antibiotic treatment required for each site and the microorganisms involved.

1.2.4 Definition of healthcare-associated infections

In our survey, we will adopt the definition of IAS proposed and updated by the CTIINILS in 2007 [18]:

"An infection is said to be associated with care if it occurs during or at the end of a patient's care (diagnostic, therapeutic, palliative, preventive or educational), and if it was neither present nor incubating at the start of the care.

When the state of infection at the start of treatment is not known precisely, a period of at least 48 hours or longer than the incubation period is commonly accepted to define a HCAI. However, it is recommended that the plausibility of the association between the treatment and the infection be assessed in each case.

For surgical site infections, infections occurring within 30 days of the operation or, if an implant, prosthesis or prosthetic device is used, within one year of the operation, are usually considered to be associated with care. However, regardless of the delay, it is recommended that the plausibility of the association between the operation and the infection be assessed in each case, taking into account the type of germ involved...".

An IN is an HCAI contracted in a healthcare establishment.

In our survey we will be targeting 5 types of nosocomial infection:

- Urinary tract infections
- Pneumopathies
- Surgical site infections
- Bacteria
- Catheter infections

Specific definitions for each infection site are given in the appendix.

1.2.5 Organisation and conduct of the study (practical arrangements for data collection)

The data will be collected by two trained interviewers.

A pre-survey of 4 to 5 days is planned to validate the questionnaire, to detect any shortcomings and to train the investigators in data collection in order to ensure that the survey itself runs smoothly.

Newly admitted patients will be included progressively, from the start date of the survey (midnight onwards).

A standardised individual form containing the patient's general information will be filled in systematically for all patients newly admitted to the department concerned.

The data will then be actively collected, with investigators visiting the department on a daily basis to detect any new cases of NI.

The new admissions list and the updated list of leavers will be consulted every day.

Information relating to hospital-acquired infections will be collated from medical

records, medical prescription forms and clinical monitoring forms (placards). Additional information may be gathered by interviewing medical or paramedical staff. The nosocomial nature of the infection will be confirmed by the treating physician, with reference to the specific definitions for each site of infection.
The date of diagnosis of an IN will be the date of onset of clinical signs.
Once the patient has been identified as having contracted an infection of the liver, a second form containing information specific to this infection will be completed.
The bacteriological data for each infection site identified will be collated from the antibiograms issued by the bacteriology laboratory.
The form will be validated systematically to ensure that it is complete.
Data collection will be limited to the predefined period of the survey and will not be continued beyond this period, even for patients who are still infected at the end of the survey.
The departments being surveyed will be informed of the aims of our survey and the practical arrangements for carrying it out, as well as the period during which it will be carried out. One or two referents (supervisor, resident) in each department will be designated to assist the investigators if they need additional information and to facilitate their tasks.

1.2.6 Indicator calculation methods

Measuring incidence requires the determination of a numerator Nt and a denominator Dt. The index t refers to the observation period.
In the calculations, the observation periods are the same for the numerator and denominator.
In our work, we will use 3 epidemiological indicators:

- Cumulative impact
- Incidence density (or incidence rate)
- The medical device exposure ratio (REDM)

We are going to calculate the overall CI and DI (all infectious sites combined) and the specific DI (according to the site of the infection, the invasive procedure, etc.).

⇨ Calculating the incidence of NI

> Cumulative impact

This is a proportion that measures risk. It is calculated by dividing the number of new cases of IN identified during the study period by the number of patients at risk of contracting an IN during the same period.
- Global

We can calculate the overall CI :

- of infected patients

o in the numerator: the number of patients with at least one infection o in the denominator: the number of patients monitored (at risk)

- infections

o in the numerator: all infections collected (all sites combined) o in the denominator: the number of patients monitored (at risk)

Overall CI of NI for the entire study population :

$$= \frac{\begin{array}{c}\textbf{nombre de nouveaux cas d'IN (tous sites confondus)}\\ \textbf{durant la periode d'étude}\end{array}}{\begin{array}{c}\textbf{nombre total de patients exposées au risque d'IN(hospitalisés} \geq \textbf{48H)}\\ \textbf{durant la même periode}\end{array}} X\ 100$$

$$\frac{\begin{array}{c}\text{number of new ND cases (all sites combined)}\\ \text{during the study period}\end{array}}{\begin{array}{c}\text{total number of patients at risk of DI (hospitalised for > 48 hours)}\\ \text{during the same period}\end{array}}$$

Example: CI of new infections (or infected patients) per 100 hospitalised patients.

- Special

For a given site of infection and a sub-population exposed to the risk of infection at this specific site (exposed to a given invasive device), we will calculate the specific CI:

Specific CI for a given infectious site:

$$= \frac{\begin{array}{c}\textbf{nombre de nouveaux cas d'infections pour ce site infectieux}\\ \textbf{chez les patients exposés durant une periode donnée}\end{array}}{\begin{array}{c}\textbf{nombre de patients exposés au risque de ce type d'infections}\\ \textbf{durant la meme periode}\end{array}} X\ 100$$

$$\begin{array}{c}\text{number of new cases of infection for this infectious site}\\ \text{in patients exposed during a given period}\\ \text{number of patients exposed to the risk of this type of infection}\\ \text{during the same period}\end{array}$$

Examples:

IC of surgical site infections per 100 surgical patients.

IC of urinary tract infections per 100 catheter patients.

IC of pulmonary infections per 100 patients Ventilators/intubes.

> Incidence density DI

It is calculated by dividing the number of new cases of infected patients occurring during a given period by the total time patients were exposed to the risk during that same period.

The length of time a patient is exposed to the risk is assessed as follows:

- For non-infected patients:

Total duration of exposure up to :

- Discharge: i.e. the length of stay on the ward (or the end of exposure to the risk in the case of a specific infection).
- Death
- Or the end of the observation period.

- For infected patients:

Length of exposure prior to the first infection (date separating the date of diagnosis of the infection and the date of admission to the department).

The time unit chosen can be the day, week or month.

> Global

Overall DI of NI for the entire study population

$$= \frac{\text{nombredenouveauxcasd'IN(ayanteuunouplusieursépisodesinfectieux)} \atop \text{toussitesconfondusdurantlaperiodeded'étude}}{\text{lasommedesduréesd'expositionsdetouslespatients} \atop \text{(infectésetnoninfectés) (enjours)}} \text{X 100}$$

number of new cases of infection (with one or more episodes of infection)
allconfusedsitesduringthestudyperiod
the duration of exposure for all patients
(infected and uninfected) (in days)

Example: DI of infected patients per 100 days of hospitalisation.

> Specifics

There are two ways of thinking about specific ID:

- <u>By site of infection</u>

Specific DI for a given infectious site :

$$= \frac{\text{nombre de nouveaux cas d'infections par site d'infection} \atop \text{pendant une periode donnée}}{\text{la somme des duréesd'expositions au risque d'infection de ce site} \atop \text{de tous les patients(infectés et non infectés) (en jours)}} \text{X 100}$$

number of new cases of infection by site of infection
during a given period

---

the sum of the durations of exposure to the risk of infection for this site
of all patients (infected and non-infected) (in days)

Note that :

s The exposure period for infected patients corresponds to the exposure period until the development of this type of infection.

- <u>By invasive procedure</u>

For a given invasive procedure (CVC, mechanical ventilation/intubation, urinary catheterisation, etc.), we will calculate the specific ID per DM:

> <u>IU on vesical survey</u> :

DI of urinary tract infections on bladder catheterisation

$$= \frac{\text{Nombre de nouveaux cas d'IU sur sonde vésicale} \atop \text{durant une période donnée}}{\text{Somme des durées d'expositions de tous les patients (infectés et noninfectés)} \atop \text{ayant été sondé vésicalement (enjours)}} \text{X 100}$$

Number of new cases of UTI on bladder catheter
during a given period

Sum of exposure times for all patients (infected and uninfected)
who have been catheterised (days)

Example: DI of urinary tract infections per 100 days of catheterisation.

^ <u>Pneumonia on mechanical ventilation (MV)/intubation</u> :

DI of respiratory infections on mechanical ventilation/intubation

$$= \frac{\text{Nombre de nouveaux cas de pneumonie sur ventilation mécanique ou intubation durant une période donnée}}{\text{Somme des duréesd'expositions de tous les patients (infectés et non infectés) ayant été ventilés mécaniquement ou intubés (enjours)}} \text{ X } 100$$

Number of new cases of pneumonia following mechanical ventilation or intubation
during a given period

Sum of exposure times for all patients (infected and non-infected)
who have been mechanically ventilated or intubated (days)

Example: DI of pneumonia over 100 days of mechanical ventilation.

> Bacteria from central venous catheterisation:

DI of bacteria on HVAC

$$= \frac{\text{Nombre de nouveaux cas de bactériémie sur CVC durant une période donnée}}{\text{Somme des durées d'expositions de tous les patients (infectés et non infectés) ayant eu un CVC (en jours)}} \text{ X } 100$$

Number of new cases of CVC bacteremia
during a given period

Sum of exposure times for all patients (infected and non-infected)
who had a CVC (in days)

Example: DI of bacteria over 100 days of CVC.

Note that :

s The exposure duration for infected patients corresponds to the duration of exposure to the DM under study until the development of this type of infection.

s The duration of exposure for patients not infected by this type of infection (including those who have been infected by other types of infection) is equal to the total duration of exposure to the DM under study.

The medical device exposure ratio (MDER)

The REDM shows, for a given department, the proportion of hospital days during which patients were exposed to a given DM.

The method used to calculate this ratio is as follows:

$$\frac{\text{La somme des journées d'exposition à un DM (cathétérisme, sondage vésical ...)}}{\text{Somme des durées de séjour des patients exposés à ce DM}} \text{ X } 100$$

The sum of days of exposure to a DM
(catheterism, bladder catheterisation, etc.)
Sum of lengths of stay for patients exposed
to this DM

Example: Ratio of exposure to a central venous catheter in intensive care.

▪=> Calculation of the medical cost of NI

To assess the cost of NI, we will look at direct medical costs. It will be presented by :

- expenditure related to the length of hospital stay, which will be determined by comparing the length of stay of a group of infected patients (cases) with another group of non-infected patients (controls).

- as well as the expenditure linked to the consumption of ATBs required by these infections. In order to estimate this additional cost, we will calculate the:

> Overall cost of extending the length of stay

Calculation of the additional cost, linked to the additional length of stay, will be based on the unit price of a day's hospitalisation, which is fixed at a flat rate by the health establishment. In estimating this cost, we will be thinking in terms of infected patients and not in terms of episodes or infectious sites, in order to simplify the calculation.

<u>Overall cost of extending the length of stay</u>

Number of infected patients *median additional length of stay *unit cost (per patient and per hospital day price)

unit cost (per patient and per hospital day)

<u>Average cost per infected patient per day</u>

Overall cost of extending length of stay

number of infected patients

> Overall cost related to the use of ATBs required by the IN

It consists of calculating the extra cost of the antibiotic treatment required for the infection. To do this, we will use data from the HCN's internal pharmacy to provide us with unit prices for 1 gram of each molecule, taking into account the routes of administration.

We will calculate two types of indicator:

<u>Average cost of ATB use per infected patient :</u>

1. For each infected patient, we will calculate the additional cost associated with the use of ATBs on a case-by-case basis using the following formula:

For each molecule of ATB consumed by a given infected patient :

Daily dose of the ATB molecule * Duration of consumption (in days)* Unit price of the molecule (in g/ml)

2. Then add up all the costs of the ATBs required for each patient
3. Then add up all the infected patients to obtain the overall cost of consumption of ATBs by infected patients during the observation period of our study.
4. Divide this overall cost by the number of infected patients to obtain the average cost of using ATBs per infected patient.

<u>Average cost of using specific ATBs for each type of infectious site:</u>

We will calculate this specific cost for the two most frequent infectious sites.

1. For each patient with the infection under study, we will calculate the extra cost of the TBA consumption required for this type of infection, using the formula given above.
2. Then add up the cost of all infectious episodes of this type of infection to give the overall cost of TBA consumption required for this type of infection.
3. Divide this overall cost by the total number of infectious episodes recorded for this type of infection to obtain the average cost of using specific ATBs for this infectious site.

1.2.7 Data management and statistical analysis

1.2.7.1 Management tools

The data will be entered, tabulated and analysed using IBM SPSS statistics software version 23.0.

1.2.7.2 Statistical analysis plan

> Descriptive section

Description of the population studied in the departments surveyed :

Breakdown of patients by: gender, age group, social security coverage, extrinsic and intrinsect risk factors, initial infection status ....

> Analytical part

A. Incidence of NI

❖ IC of infected patients:

- Global
- Special

❖ DI of infected patients

- Global
- Special

B. Risk factors for NI

The variable to be explained (dependent) will be the occurrence of nosocomial infection and the explanatory variables will be all the risk factors (intrinsic and extrinsic) collected.

Two qualitative variables will be compared using the Chi-squared test or Fisher's exact test. For quantitative variables we will use the Student's T test or the Mann Whitney U test.

We will be using :

- In the first stage: a univariate (binary) analysis to study the association between each separate risk factor and the occurrence of NI. Then, depending on the results of this first stage, we will select all the risk factors found to be significantly associated with the occurrence of NI, tolerating a significance threshold of up to 0.25. The strength of the association between the risk factors and the occurrence of infection will be measured by the crude relative risk (RR) and its 95% confidence interval.
- Secondly, all these factors will be introduced into a multivariate logistic regression model, in order to eliminate all possible confounding factors with a fixed significance level of 0.05. The adjusted RRs will then be calculated, along with their 95% confidence intervals.

C. Estimated additional cost of NI

- Additional costs associated with extending the length of stay
- Extra cost of TBA consumption

1.2.8 Ethical considerations

The survey protocol will be submitted to the HCN Ethics Committee for approval before the survey can be carried out in the field.

The information and informed consent of each eligible patient will be ensured before they are included in our survey.

2. Questionnaire for a survey on the incidence of healthcare-associated infections at Charles Nicolle Hospital in Tunis

General information

- Name and surname of the investigator :
- Patient's full name :
- Inpatient department : surgery A ☐ surgery B ☐ medical intensive care

☐

- Inpatient unit: inpatient ☐ intensive care ☐
- Patient number:
- Date of admission to hospital: |_| |_|/|_| |_|/|_|_| |_|
- Date of admission to the department: : |_| |_|/|_|_|/|_|_|_|_|
- Number of beds: Room no. :
- Gender: Female ☐ Male ☐
- Age (in years) :
- Social security coverage: indigent ☐ CNAM ☐ Payant ☐
- Transfer of patient from one department to another: yes ☐ **no^**
- Transferring a patient from one hospital to another: yes!
- Reason for hospitalisation :

Intrinsic determinants

- Mac CABE severity score: (on admission) :

0: no illness or non-fatal illness ☐

1 fatal disease within 5 years ☐

2 : rapidly fatal disease within a year ☐

3 :**unknown^**

- Diabetes : yes ☐ no ☐

if yes: Type: type I ☐ type II ☐

- HTA : or ☐ no ☐
- Respiratory failure chronic: (e.g. COPD) yes ☐ no ☐
- Smoking : yes ☐ no ☐

- *Immunodepression : yes ☐ no ☐
- Progressive neoplasia : yes ☐ no ☐
- Alcohol : yes ☐ no ☐
- Trauma : yes ☐ no ☐

Extrinsic factors

Invasive devices and procedures

- Urinary catheter: yes ☐ no ☐

Insertion date: |_|_|/|_|/|_| |_|_| Removal date: |_|_|/|_|/|_|_|
Total insertion time: |_|_| **days**

- Peripheral vascular catheter: yes ☐no ☐

Insertion date: |_|/|_|/|_| |_|_| Removal date: |_|/|_|/|_|_| Total insertion time: |_|_| **days**

- Central vascular catheter: yes ☐ no ☐

Insertion date: :|_|_|/|_|/|_| |_|_| Removal date: |_|_|/|_|/|_|_|
Total insertion time: |_|_| **days**

- Intubation: yes ☐ no ☐

Insertion date : |_|_|/|_|/|_| |_|_| Removal date : |_|_|/|_|/|_|_|
Total insertion time : |_|_| **days**

- Mechanical ventilation: yes ☐ no ☐

Insertion date : |_|_|/|_|/|_| |_|_| Removal date : |_|_|/|_|/|_|_|
Total insertion time : |_|_| **days**

- Gastric tube: yes ☐ no ☐

Date of insertion : |_|_|/|_|/|_| |_|_| Date of removal :
|_|_|/|_|/|_|_|_|_|
Total insertion time: |_||_| days

- Parental nutrition: yes □no □

Date of insertion :
Removal date: |_| |_|/|_| |_|/|_| |_||_| Total insertion time: |_||_| days

- Endoscopy: yes □no □

If yes, type
Date of action: |_| |_|/|_| |_|/|_| |_| |_|

- Drain: yes □no □

Insertion date :|_| |_|/|_| |_|/|_| |_| |_| Removal date :|_| |_|/|_| |_|/|_| |_||_| Total insertion time :|_| |_| days

- Peritoneal dialysis: yes □ no □

Date of action: |_| |_|/|_| |_|/|_| |_| |_|

- Physiotherapy: yes □ no □

Date of action: |_| |_|/|_| |_|/|_| |_| |_|

- Tracheotomy: yes □ no □

Date of action: |_| |_|/|_| |_|/|_| |_| |_|

The number of invasive devices and procedures: | _ | | _ |

Surgical intervention

In the last 30 days

- Surgery :

yes □ no □

If yes:

roperation date: LILI/LILI/LILILI

-Location:

HCN surgery department □ other □

Context :

emergency □ programmed □

-Surgical treatment :

Laparoscopic □ laparatomic □

Other □

SPECIFY:

-Type of surgery :

clean □ clean contaminated □

Contaminated □ dirty □

-Surgery time (minutes) :

During your current hospital stay

- Surgery :

yes □ no □

If yes :

-Date de roperation : LILI/LILI/LILILI

Location:

HCN surgery department □other □

Context :

emergency □ programmed □

- Length of hospital stay before the operation :

|_||_|

jo[urs]

-Surgical treatment :

Laparoscopic □ laparatomic □

Other □

SPECIFY:

-Type of surgery :

clean □ clean contaminated □

Contaminated □ Dirty □

-Surgery time (minutes) :

-surgery: simple □ complicated □

-type of **anaesthesia :**

General □ spinal anaesthesia □

Locoregionale □ local □

If general: intubation: yes □ no^

Antibiotic prophylaxis: yes □ no □ If yes:

Preoperative^ Induction of anaesthesia □

During the operation □ Post operative □

Number of molecules :

Please specify:

molecules	duration	Number of doses
1)	>=24h <24h	
2)	>=24h <24h	
3)	>=24h <24h	

*ASA score: 1 □ **20 30**

*NNIS score: 1 □ **20 30**

Initial infectious state of the patient

-Is it infected on admission to the ward? yes □ no □

If yes: type of infection: - Community **0**

- Infection contracted in another establishment/department or from another department in the same establishment □

-If infection contacted from another establishment/department: site of infection :

- Presence of a germ: yes **0** no **0**

If yes: antibiotic administered :

Has the patient become infected during the current hospitalisation?

yes **0** no **0**

If no: release date: |_|_|/|_|_|/|_|_|_|_|_|

If yes :

IAS sheet (V)re

- Date of start of diagnosis of HCAI: 1_11_1/1_11_1/1_11_11_1
- Type of infection :

o pneumonia □if yes :

was he intubated before the infection? yes □ no □

o surgical site infection □ if yes: - superficial (surgical wound) □

-deep (organ/space) □

o bacteremia □if yes :

was central catheterisation performed prior to infection? yes □ no □

o urinary tract infection ☐ if yes :

was a bladder catheter inserted before the infection? yes ☐ no ☐

o catheter infection ☐ if so: -localised ☐

-septicemic ☐

Site of infection	Invasive devices
Urinary tract infection AND	Urinary catheter in place for 7 days prior to infection: **yes^** no ☐
Pneumonia AND	Mechanical ventilation and/or intubation during the 48 hours prior to infection: yes ☐ no ☐
Bacteria AND	Central venous catheter in place within 48 hours prior to infection : yes ☐ no ☐

- Bacteriological samples taken : yes ☐ no ☐

If yes :

Type of sample	Date	Result	Micro-orgasms
-Blood ☐ -Urinary ☐ -Respiratory ☐ -Wound ☐ - other ☐		Positive ☐ Negative ☐	

Anti-infectives: yes ☐ no ☐

If yes :

- The total number: |__||__|

Type of molecules	Start date	Dosage	Duration	Type of treatment	Route of administration
1/				Empirical ☐ Targete ☐	IM □IV ☐ Oral ☐ Subcutaneous ☐
2/				Empirical ☐ Targete ☐	IM □IV ☐ Oral ☐ Subcutaneous ☐
3/				Empirical ☐	IM □IV ☐

				Targete ☐	Oral ☐
					Subcutaneous ☐
4/				Empirical ☐ Targete ☐	IM □IV ☐ Oral ☐ Subcutaneous ☐
5/				Empirical ☐ Targete ☐	IM □IV ☐ Oral ☐ Subcutaneous ☐
6/				Empirical ☐ Targete ☐	IM □IV ☐ Oral ☐ Subcutaneous ☐

Did the patient receive ATB treatment before the onset of the infection? or O **no^.**

If yes :

Start date	Dosage	Duration	Route of administration	Indication
			IM □IV ☐ Oral ☐ Subcutaneous ☐	Curative ☐ Antibioprophylactic^
			IM □IV ☐ Oral ☐ Subcutaneous^	Curative ☐ Antibioprophylactic ☐

- The total number of IAS: |_||_|

Discharge arrangements:

o Decede ☐

o Leaving with treatment^ if yes: which treatments :

Molecules	Dosage	Duration	Route of administration
1/			IM □IV ☐ Oral ☐ Subcutaneous^
2/			IM □IV ☐ Oral ☐

			Subcutaneous^
3/			IM □IV ☐ Oral ☐ Subcutaneous^

o Leaving without treatment ☐

o Transfere: ☐ o Other: □ Specify:

Main diagnosis :

Total hospital stay (in days) :

IAS acquisition period: /_//_/ days

Release date: /_//_//_//_//_//_//_/_/_/

VII. Conclusions and recommendations

HAIs are a major public health problem worldwide. They are responsible for a fairly high burden of morbidity and mortality, with a considerable economic cost in terms of treatment.

The rate of these infections is an important indicator of the quality and safety of care.

In the face of this scourge, prevention remains the most effective weapon by acting on the avoidable proportion of these infections.

Although the studies carried out on this subject are limited in our country, we can conclude that this is a serious problem which is constantly on the increase and which requires the implementation of an effective national strategy to combat these infections.

An appropriate framework for this fight is the nosocomial infection control committee (CLIN), which must be set up in each health establishment. It must be made up of a multidisciplinary team (clinicians, microbiologists, infectiologists, epidemiologists, hygienists, pharmacists, paramedical staff and administrative managers). It meets at least 3 times a year. Its role is to organise, plan and lead the fight against HCAIs in healthcare establishments, working closely with decision-makers. This committee must be associated with an operational hospital hygiene team (EOHH) responsible for implementing the action programme to combat HCAIs.

It is essential to set up a surveillance system and an internal training programme for healthcare staff in each health establishment on preventing the risk of infection. Nursing staff are a key link in the transmission of nosocomial infections. Thus, the fight against HCAI can be effective with simple gestures, especially with regard to compliance with asepsis rules and hand hygiene, which have shown their effectiveness in significantly reducing the risk of infection in hospitals. Against this backdrop, the WHO took the initiative of launching a "clean care is safer care" programme in 2005, aimed at reducing the incidence of HCAIs.

In addition to complying with hygiene and asepsis rules, understanding the underlying epidemiology of antibiotic resistance is a vital and crucial step towards formulating interventions to control its emergence and transmission in humans. Rational prescribing of antibiotics is the only way to limit the transmission of multi-resistant bacteria (MRB).

In Tunisia, a national plan to combat the emergence of BMRs (2019-2023) has recently been implemented, with recommendations.

There is no national programme to combat HCAIs, and no regulatory framework in Tunisia. There is a legal vacuum as regards the obligation to report IAS. The development of a regulatory framework would be essential not only for the implementation but also for the proper functioning of the reporting system, in order to improve the prevention of HAIs. At present, there are only simple recommendations and circulars relating to hospital hygiene activities and sanitation of the hospital and peri-hospital environment.

A law must therefore be introduced to make it compulsory for all healthcare establishments, whether public or private, to organise the fight against HCAIs.

Law no. 92-71 of 27 July 1992 on communicable diseases also needs to be revised, with HCAIs added to the list of notifiable diseases appended to the law.
Surveillance for HCAIs should now be part of the activities of healthcare establishments, which are obliged to set it up, as it will provide high-quality epidemiological data.
Finally, control, monitoring and accountability of hygiene practices must be carried out on a regular basis to reduce the occurrence of HCAIs in the hospital environment.
In conclusion, an effective programme to combat HCAI must include :

- training for care staff
- staffing
- equipment: in particular the provision of water points and appropriate equipment in sufficient quantities
- drawing up, posting, applying and supervising care and hygiene protocols and monitoring nosocomial infections, including feedback.

These recommendations can only be effective and efficient if there is a broad consensus in the organisation of care and strong support for them from staff.

References

[1] C. A. Umscheid, M. D. Mitchell, J. A. Doshi, R. Agarwal, K. Williams, and P. J. Brennan, "Estimating the proportion of healthcare-associated infections that are reasonably preventable and the related mortality and costs", *Infect Control HospEpidemiol,* vol. 32, no. 2, pp. 101-114, Feb. 2011, doi: 10.1086/657912.
[2] Allegranzi B, BagheriNejad S, Combescure C, Graafmans W, Attar H, Donaldson L, et al. Burden of endemic health-care-associated infection in developing countries: systematic review and meta-analysis. Lancet Lond Engl. 2011;377(9761):228-41. DOI: 10.1016/S0140- 6736(10)61458-4.
[3] Murni IK, Duke T, Kinney S, Daley AJ, Soenarto Y. Reducing hospitalacquired infections and improving the rational use of antibiotics in a developing country: an effectiveness study. ArchDis Child. 2015;100(5):454-9. DOI: 10.1136/archdischild-2014-307297.
[4] Arefian H, Hagel S, Heublein S, Rissner F, Scherag A, Brunkhorst FM, et al. Extra length of stay and costs because of health care-associated infections at a German university hospital.Am J Infect Control. 2016. https://doi.org/10.1016/j.ajic.2015.09.005
[5] CDC. National and State Healthcare-Associated Infections progress report. 2016. Available at: http://www.cdc.gov/HAI/pdfs/progress-report/hai-progress- report.pdf.)
[6] ECDC. Economic evaluations of interventions to prevent healthcare-associated infections: literature review. Stockholm: ECDC. 2017.
[7] Pittet D, Allegranzi B, Boyce J. The World Health Organization Guidelines on Hand Hygiene in Health Care and their consensus recommendations. Infect Control HospEpidemiol. 2009)https://doi.org/10.1086/600379
[8] E. O. Irek, A. A. Amupitan, T. O. Obadare, and A. O. Aboderin, "A systematic review of healthcare-associated infections in Africa: An antimicrobial resistance perspective," *Afr J Lab Med*, vol. 7, n° 2, Dec. 2018, doi: 10.4102/ajlm.v7i2.796.
[9] WHO | Why a global challenge on hospital-acquired infections , *WHO*. Available at https://www.who.int/gpsc/background/fr/ (consulted on July 13, 2020.
[10] ZikriaSaleem et al. Point prevalence surveys of health-care-associated infections: a systematic review .2019;113(4);191-205. Available at https://www.ncbi.nlm.nih.gov/pmc/articles/PMC6758614/ (consulted on July 13, 2020).
[11] Annabi Attia T, Dhidah L, Hamza R, Kibech M, Lepoutre-Toulemon A. Premiere enquete nationale tunisienne de prevalence de l'infection nosocomiale: principaux resultats. Tunis Med. 2007;15:144-149.
[12] Hajer LETAIEF ep MRAD. Etude de la prevalence et des facteurs de risque des infections nosocomiales en Tunisie:Resultats de l'enquete nationale 2012 [thesis]; 2017,215.
[13] A. *Jamoussiet al.*, "The prevalence of healthcare-associated infection in medical intensive care units in Tunisia. Results of the multi-centre nosorea1 study", *Tunis Med,* vol. 96, n° 10-11, pp. 731-736, Nov. 2018.
[14] 100 recommendations for the surveillance and prevention of nosocomial infections .86. available a :

https://webcache.googleusercontent.com/search?q=cache:pP4QrNef71cJ:https:// solidarites-
sante.gouv.fr/IMG/pdf/100_recommendations.pdf+&cd=1&hl=en&ct=clnk&gl=tn (consulted on July 14, 2020).

[15] Talaat M, El-Shokry M, El-Kholy J, et al. National surveillance of health care-associated infections in Egypt: developing a sustainable program in a resourcelimited country. Am J Infect Control. 2016;44(11):1296-1301.

[16] O. *Ezziet al*, Perceptions of a healthcare-associated infection reporting system in a Tunisian university hospital , *Sante Publque,* vol. Vol. 29, No. 1, pp. 115-123, March 2017, Accessed: Jul 14, 2020. [Online]. Available from: https://www.cairn.info/revue-sante-publjque-2017-1-page-115.htm.

[17] IPSE. Improving Patient Safety in Europe TechnicalImplementation Report 2005-2008 . November 2008. Available at : https:// ecdc.europa.eu/sites/portal/files/media/en/ healthtopics/Healthcare-associated_infections/ HAI-Net/Documents/healthcare-associatedinfections-IPSE-Technical-Report.pdf

[18] Reilly J, Stewart S, Allardice G, et al. Evidence-based infection control planning based on national healthcare-associated infection prevalence data. Infect Control HospEpidemiol. 2009;30(2):187-189.

[19] Surveillance of nosocomial infections: H. Sax and D. PittetRev Med Suisse 2000; volume -4. 20467

[20]Zingg W, Huttner BD, Sax H, et al. Assessing the burden of healthcare-associated infections through prevalence studies: what is the best method? 1.Infect Control HospEpidemiol. 2014

[21] Zarb P, Coignard B, Griskeviciene J, et al. The European Centre for Disease Prevention and Control (ECDC) pilot point prevalence survey of healthcare-associated infections and antimicrobial use. Euro Surveill. 2012

[22] Kepenekli E, Soysal A, Yalindag-Ozturk N, et al. A national point-prevalence survey of pediatric intensive care unit-acquired, healthcare-associated infections in Turkey. Jpn J Infect Dis. 2015

[23] Gastmeier P, Sohr D, Rath A, et al. Repeatedprevalence investigations on nosocomial infections for continuous surveillance. J Hosp Infect 2000

[24] Glenister H. Sensitivity and specificity of surveillance methods. BaillieresClin Infect Dis. 1996

[25] Geffers C, Baerwolff S, Schwab F, et al. Incidence of healthcare-associated infections in high-risk neonates: results from the German surveillance system for very-low-birthweight infants. J Hosp Infect. 2008

[26] J. M. Leoncio, V. F. de Almeida, R. A. P. Ferrari, J. D. Capobiango, G. Kerbauy, and M. T. G. M. Tacla, "Impact of healthcare-associated infections on the hospitalization costs of children," *Rev Esc Enferm USP,* vol. 53, p. e03486, August 2019, doi: 10.1590/S1980-220X2018016303486.

[27] Angelis G, Murthy A, Beyersmann J, Harbarth S. Estimating the impact ofhealthcare-associated infections on length of stay and costs. Clin

MicrobiolInfect2010;16:1729-35.
[28] hayetKammoun.infection associe aux soins definitions:hygiene hospitaliere et lute contre les infections associes aux soins.2009.p.5-9.
[29] S. Selwyn, 'SIR JOHN PRINGLE: HOSPITAL REFORMER, MORAL PHILOSOPHER AND PIONEER OF ANTISEPTICS', *Med. Hist.* vol. 10, n° 3, p. 266-274, July 1966, doi: 10.1017/S0025727300011133.
[30] Semmelweis IF. The etiology, the concept and the prophylaxis of childbed fever. Pest, CA Hartleben'sVerlag-Expedition, 1861.
[31] Celine LF. The life and work of Philippe Ignace Semmelweis. These pour le doctorat en medecine, 1936
[32] E. Ellenberg, L'infection nosocomiale : relire l'histoire et penser au présent , Sante Publique, vol. Vol. 17, no 3, p. 471-474, 2005, Accessed: July 17, 2020. [Online]. Available at: https://www.cairn.info/revue-sante-publique-2005-3- page-471.htm
[33] UVMaF Pedagogical Editorial Committee. Hygiene hospitaliere.2011 [online]. Availablea : http://campus.cerimes.fr/maieutique/UE-sante-publique/hygiene hospitaliere/site/html/1.html?fbclid=IwAR35EPV5ycgZEVbwETzJuUTh1cuxIETBCfw9zdhscqt81QbR9jTcer3FaHQ#:~:text=According%20to%20the%20committee%C3%A9%20of%20the%20ministers,care%20that%20y%20a
[34] "Ministere de la sante, de la jeunesse et des sports. Comite technique des infections nosocomiales et des infections liees aux soins". https://webcache.googleusercontent.com/search?q=cache:bQN3WDkBGFsJ:https://solidarites-sante.gouv.fr/IMG/pdf/rapport_vcourte.pdf+&cd=1&hl=en&ct=clnk&gl=tn (consulted on July 16, 2020).
[35] Daniau Come, Leon Lucie, Berger-Carbonne Anne. Enquete nationale de prevalence des infections nosocomiales et des traitements anti-infectieux en etablissements de sante, mai-juin 2017.2019, p. 270.
[36] "WHO - Promoting the rational use of medicines saves lives and money , *WHO*. https://www.who.int/mediacentre/news/notes/2004/np9/fr/ (consulted on July 13, 2020).
[37] "Antibiotic resistance". https://www.who.int/fr/news-room/fact-sheets/detail/antibiotic-resistance (consulted on July 13, 2020).
[38] S. Ali *et al*, "Healthcare associated infection and its risk factors among patients admitted to a tertiary hospital in Ethiopia: longitudinal study", *Antmicrob. Resist. Infect. Control*, vol. 7, no. 1, p. 2, Dec. 2018, doi: 10.1186/s13756-017-0298-5.
[39] P. Rattanaumpawan and V. Thamlikitkul, "Epidemiology and economic impact of health care-associated infections and cost-effectiveness of infection control measures at a Thai university hospital", *Am. J. Infect. Control*, vol. 45, n° 2, pp. 145-150, Feb. 2017, doi: 10.1016/j.ajic.2016.07.018.
[40] D. N. Pestourie, Microorganisms responsible for IAS , p. 23. available at: https://www.cpias-nouvelle-aquitaine.fr/wp-content/uploads/2017/11/1-micro-

organisme-ias.pdf
[41] R. Hamza, "EPIDEMIOLOGIE DES INFECTIONS ASSOCIEES AUX SOINS HEALTHCARE ASSOCIATED INFECTIONS EPIDEMIOLOGY", p. 4, 2010.
[42] "Infections nosocomiales", *Inserm - La science pour la sante.* https://www.inserm.fr/information-en-sante/dossiers-information/infections-nosocomiales (consulted on July 13, 2020).
[43] A. Chatterjee *et al*, "Quantifying drivers of antibiotic resistance in humans: a systematic review", *Lancet Infect. Dis*, vol. 18, n° 12, pp. e368-e378, Dec. 2018, doi: 10.1016/S1473-3099(18)30296-2.
[44] O'Neill J. Tackling drug-resistant infections globally: final report and recommendations the review on antimicrobial resistance. London: Wellcome Trust; 2016)
[45] H. Ridha, K. Hayet, and D. Mahmoud, "le risque infectieu en milieu de soin", p. 158.
[46] Scientific report of the 2016 World Consumer Rights Day "Food without ATBs" or "On the use of ATBs". p. 26, 2016.
[47] S. Carle, "Antibiotic resistance: a public health issue", vol. 42, p. 16, 2010.
[48] A. S. Ouedraogo, H. Jean Pierre, A. L. Banuls, R. Ouedraogo, and S. Godreuil, "Emergence and spread of antibiotic resistance in West Africa: contributing factors and threat assessment," *Medecine Sante Trop,* vol. 27, no. 2, pp. 147-154, May 2017, doi: 10.1684/mst.2017.0678.
[49] "L'Antibio-Resistance en Tunisie LART Données 2012- 2013 -2014". https://webcache.googleusercontent.com/search?q=cache:q4TX3iQKEZIJ:https://www.infectiologie.org.tn/pdf_ppt_docs/resistance/1544636296.pdf+&cd=2&hl=fr&ct=clnk&gl=tn (consulted on Jul. 18, 2020).
[50] MOKHTAR Lamia. Incidence de l'infection nosocomiale et approche de son coût : Resultats d'une etude prospective dans un service de chirurgie generale [thesis]; 1998,96 .
[51] "International Nosocomial Infection Control Consortium report, data summary of 50 countries for 2010-2015: Device-associated module - ScienceDirect". https://www.sciencedirect.com/science/article/abs/pii/S0196655316308057?casa_token=OG4VKKosuxsAAAAA:yUvfn_2GVNPnY825Qe43vZJcfw3lFq2olYuBqPLfB7KMNtitK6IXi2LUURiF_HJw63iRuvWglG-zA (accessed July 14, 2020).
[52] S. Iordanou, N. Middleton, E. Papathanassoglou, and V. Raftopoulos, "Surveillance of device associated infections and mortality in a major intensive care unit in the Republic of Cyprus", BMC Infect. Dis, vol. 17, no. 1, p. 607, Dec. 2017, doi: 10.1186/s12879-017-2704-2.
[53] Surveillance of nosocomial infections in adult intensive care. Reseau rea-raisin, france, results 2012. Saintmaurice: institut de veille sanitaire. 2013. 38p.
[54] Stone PW, Braccia D, Larson E. Systematic review of economic analyses of health care-associated infections. American Journal of Infection Control. 2005;33:501-509. PubMed | Google.
[55] Brun-Buisson C, Bonmarchand G, Carlet J, Chastre J, Durocher A, Fagon JY, et

al. Risques et maitrise des infections nosocomiales enreanimation : texte d'orientation SRLF/SFAR. Reanimation 2005;14:463-71.

[56] V. D. Rosenthal et al, "Six-year multicenter study on short-term peripheral venous catheters-related bloodstream infection rates in 727 intensive care units of 268 hospitals in 141 cities of 42 countries of Africa, the Americas, Eastern Mediterranean, Europe, South East Asia, and Western Pacific Regions: International Nosocomial Infection Control Consortium (INICC) findings", Infect.
Control Hosp Epidemiol, vol. 41, no. 5, pp. 553-563, May 2020, doi: 10.1017/ice.2020.20.

[57] V. D. Rosenthal et al, "Six-year multicenter study on short-term peripheral venous catheters-related bloodstream infection rates in 246 intensive units of 83 hospitals in 52 cities of 14 countries of Middle East: Bahrain, Egypt, Iran, Jordan, Kingdom of Saudi Arabia, Kuwait, Lebanon, Morocco, Pakistan, Palestine, Sudan, Tunisia, Turkey, and United Arab Emirates-International Nosocomial Infection Control Consortium (INICC) findings," J. Infect. Public Health, p. S1876034120304135, Apr. 2020, doi: 10.1016/j.jiph.2020.03.012.

[58] "Report on the Burden of Endemic Health Care-Associated Infection Worldwide Clean Care is Safer Care". https://webcache.googleusercontent.com/search?q=cache:f-6FKBmQDmgJ:https://apps.who.int/iris/bitstream/handle/10665/80135/97892415 01507_eng.pdf%3Fsequence%3D1+&cd=2&hl=en&ct=clnk&gl=tn (consulted on July 14, 2020).

[59] A. Dramowski, A. Whitelaw, and M. F. Cotton, "Burden, spectrum, and impact of healthcare-associated infection at a South African children's hospital," J. Hosp. Infect. vol. 94, no. 4, pp. 364-372, Dec. 2016, doi: 10.1016/j.jhin.2016.08.022.

[60] N. Madani, V. D. Rosenthal, T. Dendane, K. Abidi, A. Zeggwagh, and R. Abouqal, "Health-care associated infections rates, length of stay, and bacterial resistance in an intensive care unit of Morocco: Findings of the International Nosocomial Infection Control Consortium (INICC)", Int. Arch. Med, vol. 2, no 1, p. 29, 2009, doi: 10.1186/1755-7682-2-29.

[61] I. Chouchene et al, "Incidence of infections associated with medical devices in a Tunisian intensive care unit", Sante Publique, vol. 27, no. 1, p. 69, 2015, doi: 10.3917/spub.151.0069.

[62] M. Hedfi, H. Khouni, Y. Massoudi, C. Abdelhedi, K. Sassi, and A. Chouchen, " epidemiologie des infections nosocomiales: a propos de 70 cas epidemiology of nosocomial infections: about 70 cases ", Tunis. Med, vol. 94, p. 6, 2016.

[63] L. Merzougui et al, "Nosocomial infections in the resuscitation setting: annual incidence and clinical aspects in the Service de Reanimation Polyvalente, Kairouan, Tunisia, 2014", Pan Afr. Med. J., vol. 30, 2018, doi: 10.11604/pamj.2018.30.143.13824.

64] Kallel H, Dammak H, Bahloul M, Ksibi H, Chelly H, Ben HamidaC et al. Risk factors and outcomes of intensive care unitacquired infections in a tunisian icu. Med sci Med Sci Monit 2010; 16(8):PH69-75.Google Scholar,

[65] Moreno CA, Rosenthal VD, Olarte N, Gomez WV, Sussmann O,Agudelo JG, et al. Device-Associated Infection Rate and Mortality in Intensive Care Units of 9 Colombian Hospitals: Findings of the International Nosocomial Infection Control Consortium. Infect Control Hosp Epidemiol. 2006;27(4):349-56.
[66] National Nosocomial Infections Surveillance (NNIS) System Report, data summary from January 1992 through June 2004, issued October 2004. Am J Infect Control. 2004;32:470-85.
[67] Hela Ghali et al. Incidence of adverse events associated with the peripheral venous catheter in a cardiology department, Tunisia | Cairn.info ". https://www.cairn.info/revue-sante-publique-2018-5-page-663.htm (consulted on July 14, 2020).
[68] Ogeer-Gylis JS. Nosocomial infections and antimicrobial resistance in critical care medicine. J Vet Emerg Crit Care. 2006;16:1-18.
[69] Lolom I, Deblangy C, Capelle A, Guerinot W, Bouvet E, Barry B, et al. Impact d'un programme prolonge d'amelioration continue de laqualite sur le risque infectieux lie aux catheters veineux peripheriques. Presse Med. 2009;38(1):34- 42.
[70] "Incidence and risk factors for surgical site infection after caesarean section in a Tunisian maternity hospital | Cairn.info". https://www.cairn.info/revue-sante-publique-2018-3-page-339.htm (consulted on July 14, 2020).
[71] Yokoe DS, Christiansen CL, Johnson R, Sands KE, Livingston J, Shtatland ES, *et al.* Epidemiology of and surveillance for postpartum infections. Emerg Infect Dis. 2001;7(5):837-41.
[72] Nyamogoba H, Obala A. Nosocomial infections in developing countries: cost effective control and prevention. East Afr Med J. 2002;79(8):435-41
[73] A. Laberge et al, Prevention of surgical site infections: summary document. 2014.
[74] World Health Organization. WHO recommends 29 ways to stop surgical infections and avoid superbugs. Available from: <http://www.who.int/mediacentre/news/releases/2016/recommendations- surgical-infections/en/ >.
[75] D. Rondeau and S. Bertezene, "Regards croises sur les infections nosocomiales: de la responsabilisation juridique a revaluation des couts", *Droit, Deontoiogie & Soin,* vol. 13, no. 3, pp. 296-309, Sept. 2013, doi: 10.1016/j.ddes.2013.07.002
[76] Netgen, "INFECTIONS NOSOCOMIALES: REALITE ET IMPACT", *Revue Medicaie Suisse.* https://www.revmed.ch/RMS/2000/RMS-2298/20465 (consulted on May 22, 2020.
[77] R. W. Haley, D. R. Schaberg, S. D. Von Allmen, and J. E. McGowan, "Estimating the Extra Charges and Prolongation of Hospitalization Due to Nosocomial Infections: A Comparison of Methods", *Journai of Infectious Diseases*, vol. 141, n° 2, pp. 248-257, Feb. 1980, doi: 10.1093/infdis/141.2.248.
[78] J. E. McGowan, "Cost and Benefit in Control of Nosocomial Infection: Methods for Analysis", *Rev Infect Dis*, vol. 3, n° 4, p. 790-797, July 1981, doi:

10.1093/clinids/3.4.790.
[79] P. Rattanaumpawan and V. Thamlikitkul, "Epidemiology and economic impact of health care-associated infections and cost-effectiveness of infection control measures at a Thai university hospital," *American Journai of Infection Controi*, vol. 45, n° 2, pp. 145-150, Feb 2017, doi: 10.1016/j.ajic.2016.07.018.
[80] S. Karagiannidou, T. Zaoutis, N. Maniadakis, V. Papaevangelou, and G. Kourlaba, "Attributable length of stay and cost for pediatric and neonatal central line-associated bloodstream infections in Greece," *Journai of Infection and Pubiic Heaith*, vol. 12, n° 3, pp. 372-379, May 2019, doi: 10.1016/j.jiph.2018.12.004.
[81] "72-12.pdf". Accessed: July 15, 2020. [Online]. Available at: http://scolarite.fmp-usmba.ac.ma/cdim/mediatheque/e_theses/72-12.pdf.
[82] "Evaluation du cout des infections nosocomiales dans le service de reanimation medicale du CHU de Tizi Ouzou". https://webcache.googleusercontent.com/search?q=cache:Ar7GFyeezisJ:https://dl.ummto.dz/bitstream/handle/ummto/9994/evaluation_cout_infections_nosocomiales_lydia_brahimi.pdf%3Fsequence%3D1%26isAllowed%3Dy+&cd=2&hl=fr&ct=clnk&gl=tn (consulted July 15, 2020).
[83] T. Vermeil, A. Peters, C. Kilpatrick, D. Pires, B. Allegranzi, and D. Pittet, "Hand hygiene in hospitals: anatomy of a revolution", *J. Hosp. Infect.* vol. 101, n° 4, pp. 383-392, Apr 2019, doi: 10.1016/j.jhin.2018.09.003.
[84] World Health Organization. WHO Guidelines on Hand Hygiene in Health Care. (2009).
[85] Gagne D, Bedard G, Maziade PJ. Systematic patients' hand disinfection: impact on meticillin-resistant Staphylococcus aureus infection rates in a community hospital. JHospInfect 2010;75:269-272.
[86] Pokrywka M, Feigel J, Douglas B, et al. A bundle strategy including patient hand hygiene to decrease Clostridium difficile infections. Medsurg Nurs 2014;23.
[87] Ardizzone LL, Smolowitz J, Kline N, Thom B, Larson EL. Patient hand hygiene practices in surgical patients. Am J Infect Control 2013;41:487e491.
[88] H.-J. Seo, K.-Y. Sohng, S. O. Chang, S. K. Chaung, J. S. Won, and M.-J. Choi, "Interventions to improve hand hygiene compliance in emergency departments: a systematic review," Journal of Hospital Infection, vol. 102, no. 4, pp. 394-406, August 2019, doi: 10.1016/j.jhin.2019.03.013.
[89] E. Alp and N. Damani, "Healthcare-associated infections in Intensive Care Units: epidemiology and infection control in low-to-middle income countries", *J. Infect. Dev. Ctries.* vol. 9, n° 10, pp. 1040-1045, Oct. 2015, doi: 10.3855/jidc.6832.
[90] E. Bouvet and G. Brucker, "L'isolement en pratique hospitaliere*", *Medecine Mal. Infect*, vol. 28, n° 5, Supplement 1, p. 485-491, June 1998, doi: 10.1016/S0399-077X(98)71005-4.
[91] (Ucgun I, Dagli C, Kiremitci A, Yildirim H, Ak G, Aslan S. Effects of isolation rooms on the prevalence of hospital acquired pneumonia in a respiratory ICU. Eur Rev Med Pharmacol Sci. 2013;17(Suppl 1):2-8.).
[92] Bernard Grynfogel,dir. Surveillance and prevention of healthcare-associated

infections.2010.
[93] "Transmission-Based Precautions | Basics | Infection Control | CDC", feb. 06, 2020. https://www.cdc.gov/infectioncontrol/basics/transmission-based-precautions.html (consulted on July 15, 2020).
[94] V. Hsu and F. Hospital, "Prevention of Health Care-Associated Infections," *Health Care (Don **Mils**)*, vol. 90, n° 6, p. 6, 2014.
[95] A. Laberge *et al*, *Prevention of surgical site infections: summary document.* 2014.
[96] Stone PW, Braccia D, Larson E. Systematic review of economic analyses of health care-associated infections. Am J Infect Control.2005;33(9):501-509.
[97] Burke JP. Infection control-a problem for patient safety. N Engl J Med. 2003;348(7):651.
[98] Manoukian S, Stewart S, Dancer S, et al. Estimating excess length of stay due to healthcare-associated infections: a systematic review and meta-analysis of statistical methodology. J Hosp Infect. 2018;100:222-235.
[99] Organization WH. Report on the burden of endemic health care-associated infection worldwide. 2011.)
[100] European Centre for Disease Prevention and Control (ECDC). European surveillance of healthcare-associated infections in intensive care units. ECDC HAIICU protocol V1.01 Standard and Light. Stockholm: ECDC, 2010.
[101] Vincent JL, Bihari DJ, Suter PM et al. The prevalence of nosocomial infection in intensive care units in Europe. Results of the European Prevalence of Infection in Intensive Care (EPIC) Study. EPIC International AdvisoryCommittee. Jama. 1995;274(8):639-44.
[102] World HealthOrganization (WHO). Global guidelines for the prevention of surgical infection. Geneva: WHO, 2016 [103] Rigby K, Clark RB, Runciman WB. Adverse events in health care: setting priorities based on economic evaluation. J Qual Clin Practic 1999; 19: 7-1.

Appendices

ASA score (American society of Anesthesiologists): This is a score used in anaesthesia to assess the general state of health of patients [1] (Table 1).

Table 1. ASA score classification

ASA classification	Definition	Examples
ASA 1	Patient in good health	Non-smokers, non-alcohol drinkers,...
ASA 2	Patient with mild systemic disease with no major functional limitations	Current smokers, controlled obesity...
ASA 3	Patients with severe systemic disease and significant functional limitations	Active hepatitis, premature infant.
ASA 4	Patient with a serious life-threatening systemic illness	Severe valve dysfunction, sepsis...
ASA 5	A dying patient who should not survive without surgery	-Massive trauma , multiple organ dysfunction ...
ASA 6	Patient with declared brain death whose organs are removed for donation.	

Altemeier score: a useful score for classifying surgical procedures according to the risk of contamination and postoperative infection, divided into 4 classes [2] :

1. Clean surgery: No opening of hollow viscera and no notion of contamination.
2. Contaminated clean surgery: Opening of hollow viscera with minimal contamination, minimal breach of asepsis.
3. Contaminated surgery: Contamination of intestinal contents Urogenital or biliary tract with infected bile or urine Traumatic wound less than 4 hours old
4. Dirty surgery: acute bacterial inflammation without pus

Foreign body, perforated viscera, presence of pus ...

NNIS (National Nosocomial Infection Surveillance) score: This is used to define four categories of patients according to their risk of contracting a surgical site infection (SSI) and is calculated from three variables [3]. (Table 2).

Table 2. Methods of calculating the NNIS score

Variable	Class of contamination		ASA score		Duration of operation	
Value	1 or 2	3 or 4	1 or 2	3, 4, 5, or 6	<P75	>P75
Point	0	1	0	1	0	1
NNIS score	Sum of	The number of points for each variable varies from 0 to 3.				

P75: Percentile 75 of the distribution of intervention data for the surgical procedure concerned

Mac CABE severity score [4] :

This severity index is filled in by the department's medical correspondent, who must describe the patient's situation on the day of the survey, unless the patient has an HCAI. In this case, the index should take into account the patient's condition before the HCAI.

- No illness or non-fatal illness: MC 0
- Fatal disease within 5 years: MC 1
- rapidly fatal disease within a year: MC 2 :

• unknown : MC 3

Immunodepression :

Treatment that reduces resistance to infection: immunosuppressive therapy, chemotherapy, radiotherapy, corticosteroid therapy >30 days, recent high-dose corticosteroid therapy (>5 mg/kg Prednisolone>5 days) [107].

Progressive disease: haemopathy, metastatic cancer, HIV+ with CD4 <500/mm^3

Progressive neoplasia [4]:

- Malignant disease (solid tumour or haemopathy) undergoing treatment (e.g. chemotherapy, radiotherapy or current or future surgery)
- Active neoplastic process with therapeutic abstention (e.g. chronic lymphocytic leukaemia, chronic myeloid leukaemia, low-grade malignant lymphomas);
- Metastatic cancer
- Palliative care

The different types of infection and their diagnostic criteria [5] :

SURGICAL SITE INFECTION

Superficial incisional infection (SSI-S) occurs within 30 days of the operation and the infection involves only the skin and subcutaneous tissue of the incision and at least one of the following symptoms:

- Purulent drainage, with or without laboratory confirmation, from the superficial incision.
- Organisms isolated from a fluid or tissue culture obtained aseptically from the superficial incision.
- At least one of the following signs or symptoms of infection: pain or tenderness, local swelling, redness or warmth and superficial incision is deliberately opened by the surgeon, unless the incision is negative for culture.

Diagnosis of superficial incisional SSI by a surgeon or attending physician

A deep incisional infection (SSI-D) occurs within 30 days of surgery if no implant is left in place, or within one year if the implant is in place and the infection appears to be related to the surgery and the infection involves deep soft tissue (e.g. fascia, muscle) of the incision and at least one of the following:

- Purulent drainage from the deep incision but not from the organ/space component of the surgical site.
- A deep incision opens spontaneously or is deliberately opened by a surgeon when the patient has at least one of the following signs or symptoms: fever (> 38°C), pain or localized tenderness, unless the incision is culture negative.
- An abscess or any other sign of infection involving the deep incision is found on direct examination, during the repeat operation, or by histopathological or radiological examination.

Diagnosis of a deep incisional SSI by a surgeon or attending physician.

PNEUMONIA

Two or more serial chest X-rays or CT scans with an image suggestive of pneumonia for patients with underlying cardiac or pulmonary disease, and at least one of the following (in patients without underlying cardiac or pulmonary disease, a definitive chest X-ray or CT scan is sufficient):

- fever > 38°C with no other cause;
- leukopenia (<4000 CFU / mm3) or leukocytosis (> 12 000 CFU / mm3); and at least one of the following (or at least two if clinical pneumonia only = PN 4 and PN 5):
- new appearance of purulent sputum or change in the character of the sputum (colour, odour, quantity, consistency);
- cough or dyspnea or tachypnea;
- suggestive auscultation (rales or bronchial respiratory sounds), ronchi, wheezing;
- worsening of gas exchange (for example, O2 desaturation or increased oxygen requirements or increased ventilation demand); and depending on the diagnostic method used:

a) Bacteriological diagnostic test carried out by:

- Positive quantitative culture from a sample from the lower respiratory tract (LRT), the least contaminated:
- bronchoalveolar lavage (BAL) with a threshold > 104 CFU * / ml or > 5% of the cells obtained by BAL contain intracellular bacteria on direct microscopic examination (classified in the BAL diagnostic category);
- protected brush with a threshold > 10^3 CFU / ml;
- Protected distal aspiration (PDA) with a threshold > 10^3 CFU / ml.
- Positive quantitative culture from a possibly contaminated (VRI) sample:
- Quantitative culture of an IRV sample (e.g. endotracheal aspirate) with a threshold of 10^6 CFU/ ml

b) Alternative microbiology methods :

- positive blood culture not related to another source of infection;
- Positive growth in pleural fluid culture;
- pleural or pulmonary abscess with positive needle aspiration;
- histological examination of the lungs showed signs of pneumonia;
- positive tests for pneumonia caused by viruses or specific germs (Legionella spp., Aspergillus spp., Mycobacteria, mycoplasma, Pneumocystis carinii):
- positive detection of viral antigen or antibodies from respiratory secretions (e.g. EIA, FAMA, shell vial test, PCR);
- positive direct examination or positive culture from bronchial secretions or tissues;
- seroconversion (e.g. influenza virus, Legionella spp., Chlamydia spp.);
- detection of antigen in urine (Legionella spp.).

<u>URINARY TRACT INFECTION</u>

- The patient presents with at least one of the following signs and symptoms without any other recognised cause: fever (> 38°C), urgency, frequency, dysuria or suprapubic tenderness.
- the patient has a positive urine culture, i.e. > 10^5 micro-organisms per ml of urine with no more than two species of micro-organisms.

<u>BACTERIEMIA</u>

- A positive blood culture for a recognised pathogen

or - the patient presents at least one of the following signs or symptoms: fever (> 38°C), chills or hypotension

and

- two positive blood cultures for a common skin contaminant (from two separate blood samples, usually within 48 hours).

Skin contaminants = coagulase negative staphylococci (including S. epidermidis), Micrococcus spp, Propioni bacteriumacnes, Bacillus spp, Corynebacterium spp.

Sources of blood infection:

- Catheter-related: the same micro-organism has been cultured from the catheter where symptoms improve within 48 hours of catheter removal (C-PVC: peripheral catheter, C-CVC: central vascular catheter).
- Secondary to another infection: the same micro-organism has been isolated from another site of infection, or there is strong clinical evidence that the blood infection was secondary to another site of infection, an invasive diagnostic procedure or a foreign body:

- pulmonary;
- urinary tract infection
- digestive tract infection
- surgical site infection;
- skin and soft tissue
- Other (e.g. meningitis, osteomyelitis, etc.)
- Primary bloodstream infections include catheter-related bacteremia and bacteremia of unknown origin.

A CVC-associated bloodstream infection according to CDC / NHSN definitions (different from CVC-related bacteremia) is a primary bacteremia with the use of a central vascular catheter (even intermittent) in the 48 hours prior to the onset of the infection: therefore the presence of the relevant device (central / peripheral vascular catheter) in the 48 hours prior to the onset of the infection is collected even in the absence of microbiological confirmation.

<u>CATHETER-RELATED INFECTION</u>

	HVAC	CVP
CRI1 (local infection)	(no positive blood culture) • Quantitative CVC culture > 103 CFU / ml or semi-quantitative CVC culture > 15 CFU and • pus / inflammation at the insertion site or tunnel.	(no positive blood culture) - Quantitative culture of PVC > 103 CFU / ml or semi-quantitative culture of PVC > 15 CFU and - pus / inflammation at the insertion site or tunnel
CRI2 (general infection)	(no positive blood culture) • Quantitative CVC culture > 10^3 CFU / ml or semi-quantitative CVC culture > 15 CFU and • clinical signs improve within 48 hours of catheter removal.	(no positive blood culture) - Quantitative culture of PVC > 103 CFU/ml or semi-quantitative culture of PVC > 15 CFU and - clinical signs improve within 48 hours of catheter removal.
CRI3 (infection	- Bacteria occurring 48 hours before or after	Bacteriaoccurring 48

of the blood circulation)	removal of the catheter and positive culture with the same micro-organism: - quantitative CVC culture > 10^3 CFU / ml or semi-quantitative CVC culture > 15 CFU; - quantitative ratio of blood culture CVC-blood sample / peripheral blood sample > 5 (3); - differential delay in the positivity of blood cultures: blood cultureCVC positive two hours or more before peripheral blood culture (blood samples taken at the same time); - positive culture with the same micro-organism using pus from the insertion site.	hours before or after catheter removal and positive culture with the same micro-organism: - quantitative culture of PVC > 10^3 CFU / ml or semi-quantitative culture of PVC > 15 CFU; - positive culture with the same micro-organism from the pus of the insertion site.

Comments:

- CVC = central vascular catheter; PVC = peripheral vascular catheter.
- Colonisation of the central vascular catheter should not be reported.
- A CRI3 (-CVC or -PVC) is also a bloodstream infection with the source C-CVC or C-PVC respectively; however, when a CRI3 is reported, the BSI should not be reported in the point prevalence survey; BSI related to the microbiologically confirmed catheter should be reported as a CRI3.

[1] "ASA Physical Status Classification System | American Society of Anesthesiologists (ASA)". https://www.asahq.org/standards-and- guidelines/asa-physical-status-classification-system (accessed July 15, 2020.

[2] "ISO-Raisin network Surveillance of surgical site infections Protocol nationalAnnee2010 ". https://webcache.googleusercontent.com/search?q=cache:7eeyVz1dUuEJ:https://www.santepubliquefrance.fr/content/download/143236/2123976+&cd=1&hl=en&ct=clnk&gl=tn (consulted on July 15, 2020).

[3] SPF, "Enquete nationale de prevalence 2012 des infections nosocomiales et des traitements anti-infectieux en etablissements de sante. May-June 2012. Protocole-guide de l'enqueteur". /maladies-and-traumatismes/infections- associées-aux-soins-et-resistance-aux-antibiotiques/infections-associees-aux- soins/enquete-nationale-de-prevalence-2012-des-infections-nosocomiales-et- des-traitements-anti-infectieux-en-etablissements-de-sante.-mai-... (consulted on Jul. 15, 2020.

[4] European Centre for Disease Prevention and Control, Point prevalence survey of healthcare-associated infections and antimicrobial use in European acute care hospitals: protocol version 4.3, full-scale survey and codebook. Stockholm: ECDC, 2012.

[5] "Ministry of Health, Youth and Sport. Comité technique des infections nosocomiales et des infections liees aux soins". https://webcache.googleusercontent.com/search?q=cache:bQN3WDkBGFsJ:https://solidarites-sante.gouv.fr/IMG/pdf/rapport_vcourte.pdf+&cd=1&hl=en&ct=clnk&gl=tn (consulted on July 16, 2020).

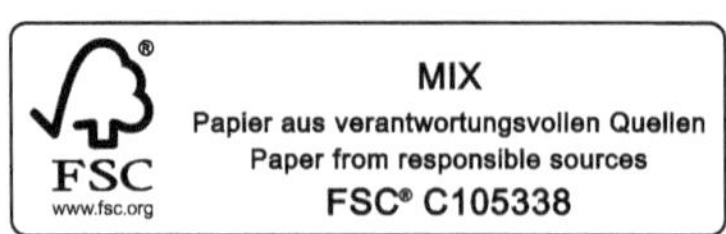

Printed by Books on Demand GmbH, Norderstedt / Germany